The Best Labour Possible?

This book is for John and Joyce Swannell, with very much love – even now, in moments of crisis, I conjugate a strong verb!

Commissioning editor: Mary Seager
Desk editor: Deena Burgess
Production controller: Chris Jarvis
Development editor: Caroline Savage
Cover designer: Helen Brockway

The Best Labour Possible?

Lesley Hobbs

BA, SRN, RMN, RN

Cartoons by Ros Asquith

Illustrations by Andy Dakin

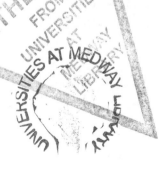

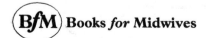

(B*f*M) Books *for* Midwives

OXFORD AUCKLAND BOSTON JOHANNESBURG MELBOURNE NEW DELHI

Books for Midwives
An imprint of Elsevier Science Limited
Robert Stevenson House
1-3 Baxter's Place
Leith Walk
Edinburgh EH1 3AF

First published 2001
Reprinted 2002
© Lesley Hobbs 2001

British Library Cataloguing in Publication Data
A catalogue record for this book is
available from the British Library

ISBN 0 7506 5200 4

Typeset by Avocet Typeset, Brill, Aylesbury, Bucks
Printed and bound in Great Britain by Biddles Ltd, Guildford and King's Lynn

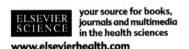

ELSEVIER SCIENCE

your source for books,
journals and multimedia
in the health sciences

www.elsevierhealth.com

Contents

Introduction

The vast majority of the changes that have occurred in childbirth over the last twenty years have been consumer-led. It is evident, however, that these changes can only be made to happen if women, at an individual level, are aware of their options and of the decisions that they can make. This book is intended to give women the information they need to make their decisions and, in this way, to effectively alter the balance so that they take a full, participating role in their own care and in the birth of their babies.

Throughout the text, the midwife is referred to in the female gender and babies in the male, to avoid clumsy repetition. I do hope that male midwives in particular will be understanding about this convention!

Acknowledgements

Yet another book which is all Henry's fault. I was going to write a bonkbuster until he persuaded me that any talent I have lies in an altogether different direction. I must thank all at BfM – their patience is little short of saintly – for waiting much too long for this, and all my friends, especially Brenda van der Kooy, who answered questions and advised me on matters of practice.

Finally, as ever, to my wonderful family, Pete, Greg, Georgia and Susannah for putting up with my snarls when it wasn't going right and my absence when it was: thank you.

1

Equal partnership in care

As humans, we often behave unpredictably and, throughout the ages, societies have formulated written and unwritten codes of behaviour to determine what is socially acceptable. Each generation modifies these social norms. With the miniskirt, society accepted that more of the human body may be shown; with co-education, society accepted that educating boys and girls together may be a positive development. It is much the same in medical/professional relationships, as other social changes are making their mark.

Women are becoming used to being in control of other facets of their lives. More women own their own homes, more women are running their own businesses. It is becoming accepted that we will not tolerate a paternalistic approach to medical care, and that an unequal relationship is detrimental to health. If we retain our autonomy, we are more likely to retain our responsibility too. This is quite a culture change within a system that has been used to dictating the delivery of its service and there will be areas where the speed of this change is faster than in others.

During your pregnancy, you should be aware that it is up to you to choose who you would like to have as your main carer – midwife, GP or obstetrician – and that you are at liberty to change your mind about where you want to have your baby, and who with, at any point, up to and including when you go into labour.

The role of each of these practitioners is different, and the relationship that you have with each will be different. Some you will meet because of and during your pregnancy only, others you may have a longer-term relationship with and may have known in other circumstances. Together, you and they form a partnership of care, with individual and collective responsibilities. It may be novel for you to see your role as one of partnership, but without you, the professionals would be without a job! You have your own responsibility within the partnership: to decide what kind of care you would like and to make decisions, according to your needs, about the professional advice you seek.

We talk a lot about 'partners' these days. Where 'partner' used to be associated with a business or professional relationship, such as those within firms of solicitors or GP practices, it is now also used to describe the person to whom we are closest, and with whom we have an intimate relationship. It is a neutral term, reflecting the acceptance within our society of sexual relationships which are not legally recognised and/or with persons of the same sex.

We think of a partnership as a shared responsibility within an association. This does not, however, absolve any of us from an individual responsibility within the partnership. It is, rather, a term which reflects the mutual interest within the association and our commitment to it.

'Partnership' is not a term that springs to mind for many women, when they consider their experience of care in childbirth, and yet that is what, essentially, concerns this book – an association or relationship between two or more parties involved in an enterprise. Partnerships are not always of an equal nature, but in the 'business' of childbirth, a satisfactory outcome is more likely when the relationship is equal and when each partner takes and has an equal and individual responsibility. A satisfactory outcome, in this context, is when all the parties feel good about the business of doing or, perhaps, having done, 'the business' (if you'll excuse the expression!).

The majority of pregnant women are likely to become involved mainly with midwives and doctors. The number of carers and depth of your involvement with them will vary according to where you live and the system of maternity services offered.

Midwives

Midwives have been around since the beginning of recorded time and are specialists in normal childbirth. Every midwife has undertaken a course which enables her to:

'...give the necessary supervision, care and advice to women during pregnancy, labour and the postpartum period, to conduct deliveries on her own responsibility and to care for the newborn and the infant.'
The Midwife's Code of Practice, 1994

The role of a midwife is defined by law and a midwife is accountable for her own practice. Whilst a midwife may care for women on her own responsibility when the circumstances are normal, she is also the principal care-giver when things are more complicated, although in these circumstances she may be carrying out treatment prescribed by an obstetrician. The midwife's skill lies in monitoring the normal, diagnosing the abnormal and making an appropriate referral when necessary.

The midwife may practise in many settings. The majority of midwives are employed by the National Health Service, and work for a Health Authority/Board or a Trust. They will work within the framework of care offered by that Trust, either in the community or in hospital.

Some midwives may also work independently of the NHS, as they prefer to work autonomously, and offer a service that can be more flexible and personal. They will offer you continuity of care throughout your pregnancy, labour and postnatally, and usually do home-births or domino deliveries.

General practitioner

Your general practitioner (GP) may be your first encounter with the system. He or she will explain their role within the process. Some GPs are more involved in maternity care than others. The GP's role today is largely confined to antenatal and postnatal care. Most GPs see maternity care as an integral part of their cradle-to-grave caring role, and feel that their knowledge of the woman and her family is valuable in this major life event in the couple's life, but the constraints on surgery time, and lack of relevant experience, means that very few GPs today will be involved with labour and birth. Some private GPs offer antenatal care, but very few will be involved with the actual delivery of your baby.

Obstetrician

Obstetrics has developed over the last two centuries, and the obstetrician is frequently the practitioner who takes overall responsibility for your care throughout the pregnancy. He or she is a doctor who has spent about ten years specialising in obstetrics and gynaecology before gaining a consultant's post. He or she may practice in and out of the NHS, so if you want private care, you may find that this is available, but at the local NHS hospital, unless you live in an area where there is a private maternity hospital. Even if you have a private obstetrician, it is unlikely that they will look after you in labour, as this care is usually provided by the midwives.

The obstetrician can give expert advice if your pregnancy is, or becomes, complicated and is usually responsible for policies and procedures within the hospital. In many parts of the country, all pregnant women are referred to an obstetrician during their pregnancy. Even if you never meet him or her, if you deliver in hospital, your care will be organised according to the protocols written by the obstetricians. This includes, for example, how many ultrasound scans are performed and when, or how long overdue you can go before induction of your labour is recommended.

The multi-disciplinary team

You may find that maternity care in your area is provided by more than one of these professionals. There is often a multi-disciplinary team, who between them provide care and expertise, and that care is usually divided between hospital and GP's surgery. Communication networks between obstetrician, GP and midwife are usually clearly defined, and referral between them is easily made.

If you have a medical condition which is relevant to your pregnancy, such as diabetes, kidney disease or heart disease, then a referral is made to the relevant specialist, who will also be involved in your pregnancy care. You may already know this specialist well and in some areas combined clinics are held, so that you don't have to make too many trips to the hospital and to make communication between the specialties easier.

Equal partnership

This new kind of relationship of equal partnership requires the development of a new set of guidelines to determine what is and is not acceptable. The concepts of choice, control and autonomy apply to all partners, but not always in equal measure. You have a choice about

- where you give birth to your baby
- who your care-giver may be
- what type of care you would like.

The medical profession has a choice about

- whether they will continue to provide their professional advice and expertise to you
- what category of care they will and can offer.

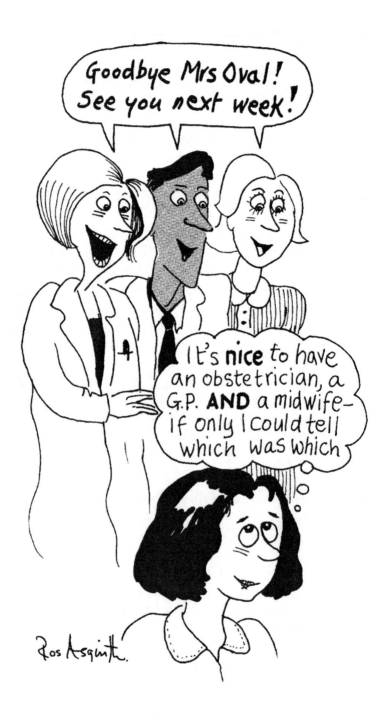

The midwife's practice is often constrained by the policies decided by the obstetricians, unless she practises independently, but she maintains her professional autonomy in the care of women experiencing normal childbirth. She is bound by law to attend you, even when her professional advice has been disregarded, so her choices are ultimately limited.

The boundaries of choice

There are always boundaries to choice; they may be geographical, ideological, ethical or practical.

Most care is organised geographically. GP practices tend to serve local areas, and few are willing to accept people who live far away. In some areas there may only be one surgery, limiting choice, and when you register, some doctors' lists may be full. You can change your GP, just for the antenatal period if, for example, you want a homebirth and your usual doctor doesn't support them.

There is usually a midwife attached to the surgery (or to a specific GP) and, in the majority of cases, opting to have her as one of your carers is both acceptable and practical. In cases where there is a problem, however, both parties have the right to exercise their choice and to request a change. If you find that there are differences of opinion, ideology or just of personality, it is not only justifiable, but also sensible, for either you or the professional to suggest a change.

Mutual respect is imperative in any partnership, and part of this is honesty and integrity. The relationship will be damaged if either of you ceases to trust the other. You have a right to clear, comprehensive, unbiased and accurate information, from all your carers, on which to base your choices.

Another constraint is financial. To provide a service that offers true choice is expensive, and there are many competing demands on public money, particularly within the NHS. The public's expectations have been consistently raised about what they should be receiving from the public sector, and arguments rage about whether the funds have been allocated to meet these expectations and the increase in demand on the services.

The heightening of public awareness and its increased requirements have put pressure on the NHS: it is expected to continue to provide all existing services, to implement new services and to operate with greater efficiency, but with no extra funding, indeed in many areas with less funding. This means, inevitably, that some services must be cut or reduced. Choices have to be made about what the priorities are, as in effect the cake is becoming smaller, and there are more slices required from it.

Changing childbirth

The Government's expert advisory group on maternity services brought out its report, *Changing Childbirth* in 1993. It called for fundamental change to the ethos of maternity care and to how maternity care services are organised. Amongst other things, it called for you to be cared for in labour by a professional whom you have come to know during your pregnancy, and makes you the focus of that care.

This has huge implications for the current system, where midwives work in fixed places. It also has cost and personnel implications, because babies can be born at any hour of the day or night, and at any point between 37 and 43 weeks of pregnancy – production control has always been a tricky point in maternity care provision! Providing you with a known midwife when you are in labour can be achieved, but it means complete reorganisation of working practices, moving midwives out of hospital into the community, making them mobile, enabling them to communicate with the women in their care and their base, and paying them for the extra hours and unsocial hours that they work. In some areas, midwives practise in teams, which can vary in number from four to twelve. Ideally you should meet all of them, so that you are always looked after by a midwife that you know, but this can make continuity of care, often an important issue for women, impossible.

Providing continuity of care is also important to midwives, but it can be very disruptive to working hours and family life. It comes at a price, and the price may be that some midwives feel unable to work like that. It may also mean that some Trusts decide that something else has to be sacrificed so that they can provide this extra service, which will not be funded in existing budgets.

Sometimes there may be a problem in the form of lack of expertise. The changes outlined in *Changing Childbirth* demand skills that may not have been developed by some practitioners working under the former, more fragmented, system. It may take time for these skills to be achieved, and in the short term, care may become even more fragmented as these practitioners are updated. Time itself is another constraint, as a pregnancy is by nature a finite period of time and it may be that these changes will not be realized before your baby is born. This shouldn't stop you being offered, and asking for, the service which is best suited to you and your new family.

The challenge for those managing the maternity services is to make the changes envisaged by *Changing Childbirth* happen, and to make them available to you and every other pregnant woman. It is easy to set limits on the provision of care; what takes imagination is the distribution of the resources available to provide a quality service for all, whilst meeting the needs of each individual.

What is important is that you, individually and collectively, make demands upon the system. Without those demands, the changes outlined above simply won't happen and women will continue to be offered the lowest common denominator of care, rather than the best of all possible options.

2

Assessing your own needs

Birth should not be a matter of luck. No matter how you have your baby, you should have good memories of your experience. So, how are you going to identify what is most important to you in terms of your pregnancy, labour, birth and into the uncharted waters of parenting this baby?

You will need to look at your own life experiences; those that have influenced you most and made you the person that you are. You will have been influenced by the people to whom you are closest. You will also have been influenced by other factors, such as exposure to the media, other people's stories and the views of the culture in which you live.

Some people find it useful to write down their ideas and influences. On any given topic (for example, what to expect in labour), you set out your ideas in one column, then set out what you have heard, where this information came from and when, in other columns and correlate it. This should give you a clearer understanding of the accuracy and provenance of your thoughts.

By looking at the influences in your life, you can understand how some of your ideas and attitudes have been formed. This will help you to identify the positive and negative feelings you have about pregnancy and birth. Look at stories you've been told about pregnancy and birth, who told you them, and whether they are important to

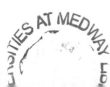

you, or even formative in your decision making. Check your impressions with other people's experiences from as wide a range as possible – you need to know how realistic they are.

We all have a level of ambivalence when contemplating what is called 'a major life event' – having a baby certainly constitutes that (coming second only to moving house, apparently!). If every woman you know has had a hospital birth or difficulties in labour, then this will make it hard for you to consider a home birth, for example, as a valid option. By identifying the issues, you will find it easier to deal with them and, in so doing, will be able to reach your decisions with confidence.

You may have limited, or no, experience of looking after a baby. You may worry that you will not be good enough as a parent or know what to do with your new baby.

You may consider how you feel about how you were parented yourself, and what you would do differently as a parent. Nobody is ever as useless as they fear they are going to be. You might even say that worrying about it is a sign that your parenting will be based upon the most fundamental good parenting precept – wanting the best for your own child. Do remember though, that part of your midwife's role is to provide you with professional advice, assistance and help, which will support you in those traumatic early days when you think that you will never, ever be able to live a normal life again!

How do you negotiate the care that you want? It will be useful to list the things that are most important to you. These will be particular to you, as individuals and as couples if you are in a partnership. Some points you might like to consider are:

- where you want to give birth
- the options available for your care
- who will support you while you are in labour

- whether you want your partner to attend antenatal visits with you and share in the decision making

- knowing the midwife who will provide your care in labour, at the birth and postnatally

- antenatal classes – are they open to your partner, the content, times, where held, by whom and any cost

- breast feeding support – who and what is available to help you to breastfeed your baby successfully.

You may find that many of your questions will be answered by your chosen carers when you first make contact and before your booking interview. You should be given information about what to expect, a description of the care and support available, or a consultation to discuss the services offered before you book for any particular form of care. Many women book for hospital delivery by default, because they don't realise that there are issues to be resolved and they find themselves 'in the system' without having given their explicit consent to it. Remember – you don't have to make decisions, about the place of birth, for example, until you feel you have explored all the options available.

You should make contact with several organisations that specialise in providing information on pregnancy, labour, birth and parenting, such as the National Childbirth Trust, the Association for Improvement in Maternity Services, the Active Birth Centre, or the Independent Midwives Association, so that when you make your final decision, you are well informed. Discuss your needs and wishes with people whose opinions you value. This may include your local community midwife, family, friends, your GP or an obstetrician.

Booking means that you have accepted a particular form of care. If you wanted to, you could go on seeing your midwife or GP at the local surgery until you have made up your mind. This will not affect your access to facilities such as scans or blood tests and will give you time to make up your mind. It is important to remember, however, that even when you have booked for a particular type of care, or even a particular carer, you can change your mind at any point, up to and including labour.

Before you attend your booking consultation, write out a list of questions to ask your midwife or obstetrician. This will make your consultation less stressful, particularly if you are attending a busy clinic, as it is often easy to forget things in an unfamiliar environment. If you are fortunate, a great deal of consideration will have been given to the needs of women (and their partners, if appropriate) coming for their first appointment. An appointment time of at least one hour is usual for your booking interview with the midwife. This will allow enough time to record your medical and obstetric history, for the checks to be done and for you to discuss particular aspects of care that are important to you. Find out before your appointment if there are crèche/childcare facilities if you have another child to consider – having a bored toddler running riot in the antenatal clinic will aid neither your concentration, nor your blood pressure.

Building trust

A degree of trust is essential to the successful outcome of your care, particularly as pregnancy and birth are at the same time the most public and the most private times of your life. Potentially difficult situations can be defused quickly if you have established a relationship built on mutual respect and trust. Your midwife and/or doctor will value your honesty, as it will help them in the provision of the right care for you. Building a relationship with your midwife may not happen on the first visit, as you will need to get to know each other and to value each other's role. Continuity of carer, (regularly seeing the same midwife, or one of a small team of midwives, who will deliver your baby), will greatly assist in building the relationship.

It is important for you to understand that any personal information about yourself or your partner should always remain confidential.

Your carers are obliged to keep all details about you confidential. Should you at any time have personal information that is particularly sensitive to you and/or you do not wish your partner to be made aware it, do tell your midwife. She will be able to advise you about whether or not it has any significance to your, or your baby's, health. She will also be able to ensure your privacy and confidentiality, even in situations where the information needs to be shared with other professionals providing you with care.

Early in 1994, and following the *Changing Childbirth* report, the Government published *The Patient's Charter, Maternity Services* which sets a guide for standards of care to be provided by the NHS. Even more importantly it sets out, specifically, the rights of the client, i.e. you. The charter clearly invites you, as a client, to take some of the responsibility for your care. A copy of the charter should be given to all women at booking, or be available in all NHS antenatal clinics. If it isn't, ask for a copy.

As mentioned previously, you do have the right to change your carers, or, indeed any of your plans, at any stage in your pregnancy. This may simply mean moving from one 'team' of carers in the hospital to another, or you may prefer to go elsewhere. If you live in or near a city, you may have the benefit of several NHS facilities within a reasonable travelling distance. Changing to another NHS hospital may mean you are unable to receive the services of their community midwives, but this may be outweighed if the care they can offer is more specific to your needs. There are also professionals who work outside the NHS who offer care tailored to individual needs. This is usually at a cost to you, but it does not mean that you will be prohibited from a hospital birth should that be your choice, or if you and/or your baby need care at a hospital.

You are entitled to get a second opinion on the proposed management of your care. You can get a referral from your midwife or GP, or it may be that you will have to seek this opinion yourself. A valuable contact would be one of the local voluntary organisations. These organisations have information on most aspects of maternity care. Even if they are unable to answer your question specifically, they will probably be able to tell you who to contact.

You should always value yourself and your feelings. Don't accept care that leaves you feeling vulnerable, or that refuses to give information, or gives information to you in a way that intimidates, confuses, or leaves you unable to make an informed choice. After all, it's you who's left holding the baby!

Dealing with problems

If you make a choice of carer and, after a period of time, you decide this is no longer appropriate to your needs, can you change? The answer is, yes, you can, but the best advice is, first talk to your midwife about what you want that isn't being realised. This will give her the opportunity to discuss the problem with you and to talk about the service offered. It will also give her the opportunity to find a solution. If she cannot help, she will be able to advise you about the person who could, and may be able to put you in touch with this person.

The Head of Midwifery Services at the local hospital, or perhaps one of the members of the obstetric team, should be available for an appointment, or they may phone, or meet you to discuss the problem. If these options are not made available to you, write to the hospital with your complaint and ask your GP or midwife for a referral elsewhere. Every hospital should advertise the appropriate line of communication for complaints, or the procedure to take the matter up for discussion with a senior member of the organisation. If the problem you find yourself faced with is causing much distress and you are feeling vulnerable, or you don't have the energy to confront the staff, try to write out an account of the situation as soon as possible.

Sometimes women feel afraid that they will be labelled as a 'bad patient', or that the staff will take 'it' out on them and the baby. This, whilst an indictment of the service, may lead to women making a formal complaint when they have had the baby, rather than at the time. When, at a later date, you feel stronger, you should inform the organisation of your grievance. If the organisation isn't aware you have a grievance, they cannot deal with it, which means that other women may have to suffer as you have.

Most problems can be resolved, given time to discuss them. Your carers will be attempting to provide the best service they can. Sometimes, in the efforts to provide that service, there will be over-sights. Most organisations make an effort to tailor care to individuals, but resources are finite; if you are unable to organise the care you want, policies change, or facilities become unavailable, look around. There may be other hospitals or individuals who will be able to help you.

Try to discuss any concerns you have calmly and in a constructive way. You will be better received if you can put your grievances across firmly, but without aggression. Being assertive, rather than aggressive, will enable you to put your concerns clearly. In order to be assertive, however, you need to understand what your rights are and how to ensure they are enforced.

3

Access to care

NHS maternity services

The National Health Service (NHS) has an obligation to provide maternity services to all women resident in the UK, including antenatal, labour and postnatal care. This takes place at home, in GP surgeries, and in institutions such as hospitals and smaller maternity units, like the former 'cottage hospitals' and 'maternity homes', now usually referred to as GP units, or community units. As explained in Chapter 1, the relevant professionals involved are midwives, GPs and obstetricians.

Although the pattern of maternity care is broadly similar throughout the UK, the way the service is delivered may vary considerably from one area to another. The size of the local population usually determines the size of the hospital and the facilities it offers, for example, specialist services such as fertility treatment, or high level neonatal care. There are often several hospitals offering maternity care in a locality, especially in large cities. In more rural areas, there may not be a choice of units, and in very remote places, such as the Scottish Islands, women may be 'bussed' to the nearest mainland unit to await the onset of labour. Where choices are restricted in this way, you should look carefully at your options, such as having your baby at home, before you make your decision.

Most women these days have their babies in hospital, but many say they aren't given a choice, not realising that they have the right to choose. It has also been reported that women are being assured of a particular system of care antenatally, only to find, when they go into labour, that they are unable to get what they had been promised. This makes asking other women, and local consumer groups, even more important. You may find it useful to keep a written record of your discussions and to confirm the assurances given in your birth plan.

Hospital consultant units

If you think that you would like to have all the personnel and equipment around just in case, then hospital is the right choice. You will go in when labour starts and be delivered by a hospital midwife, or you may be able to arrange with your community midwife that she will go with you.

If you have a choice of hospital, then there are other issues to be considered:

- How accessible is each unit?

- What is the accommodation like?

- What do other women say about each one?

- Is there a policy of active management of labour and, if so, do you want to have your labour artificially managed? (See Chapter 5 for details)

- What percentage of women already know the midwife who will attend them in labour?

- Do they routinely starve women in labour? (The research does not support this)

- Do they always put women on a fetal heart monitor? Bearing in mind that the World Health Organisation says that this is unevaluated practice and, without evidence of fetal distress, can in some cases lead to inaccurate diagnoses of fetal distress, do you want this? (See Chapter 6 for a fuller discussion.)

- Do they have a birth pool and will you be able to have the baby in it, or, alternatively, just use it for pain relief if you want to?

- Do they have an epidural service? If the answer is yes, then is it available 24 hours a day? Does the anaesthetist also cover the rest of the hospital? If so, you may have to wait for your epidural for a very long time.

- What are the statistics at the hospital on the following procedures:

- Caesarean section

- Assisted deliveries (forceps and ventouse)

- Epidurals

- Vaginal breech births

- Induction

- What is their breastfeeding rate?

You can ask for information on their policies or statistics, but many hospitals do not have, or are unwilling to produce, such information. If you strike lucky, go away to read it before you decide to book for care, but if you don't, then contact the local Community Health Council (CHC) or the trust's Maternity Services Liaison Committee (MSLC). These two organisations may well have the information, but if not, you can ask them to get it for you. All CHCs are listed in the phone book, and the name of the secretary of the MSLC can be obtained direct from the hospital or from the local branch of the National Childbirth Trust. When enough women ask for this sort of information the trusts will routinely provide it.

Make a list of the pros and cons of each hospital and decide which, on balance, best meets your needs. Then ask to be referred there.

GP unit (district hospital, or in some areas, a small cottage hospital)

These maternity units are usually available to local women and access to them is controlled by GPs. You should weigh up the advantages of a small unit against the resources at a large one and choose the option that feels right to you. Women with complicated pregnancies, or who will predictably have problem labours, are not advised to give birth at these units, but can usually transfer there for postnatal care afterwards. If there is no pool, would you be able to bring a hired one with you? Will you be encouraged to be mobile, and to use positions which help you? Do ask and, again, don't book until you are satisfied that all your queries have been addressed rather than dismissed.

You will be cared for by your community midwife, or one of her colleagues, or a midwife working at the unit. Ask about this before you book, as it may be possible to arrange for a midwife you know to look after you. You stand a good chance of having a low tech birth, but do remember that there is unlikely to be either an anaesthetist or an intensive care unit at these hospitals, so if you want an epidural, or your baby needs the services of a paediatrician, or if a problem arises, then you will have to be transferred to a consultant unit.

Home

Many women would like to give birth at home but are talked out of it. For a healthy woman, having a normal pregnancy, home is a perfectly safe option – at least as safe as hospital and with far lower risks of unnecessary intervention, or infection. There are advantages in having your own things round you and being able to eat and drink when you want to. Having professionals as guests in your house can give you a sense of control, especially if you are not fond of clinical environments. You can have the baby where you please and have the people there that you want – nobody needs to be excluded, unless you want them to be. This would include your other children, obviously.

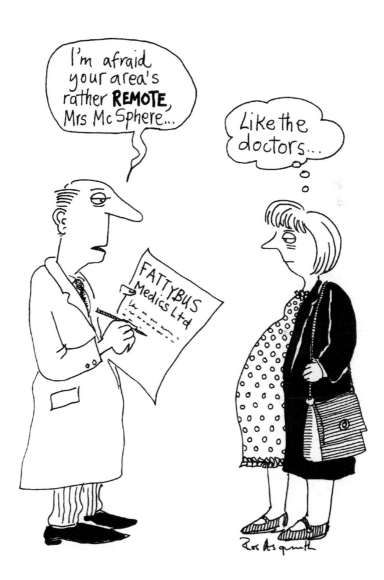

As with the small hospitals, if a problem should arise, you will need to transfer to hospital and you should include this possibility in your deliberations. You may find it helpful to read the MIDIRS *Informed Choice* leaflet[1] on the place of birth, which covers this issue.

An epidural is not an option, but other forms of pain relief such as TENS, pethidine and entonox (gas and air) are available and you can use a pool if you want to. Bear in mind that you may have to hire a pool, or a TENS machine, if your chosen unit doesn't have one and you would like to use it (see Chapter 6).

Non-NHS options

Maternity, or birth, centres

These are midwife-run, independent centres, which are usually privately funded, but may have NHS provision. They are a new development over the last few years, but bear some resemblance to the old Maternity Homes. They may be free standing, or sometimes in the grounds, or part of, a larger private hospital. At a Maternity Centre, you can have antenatal care, classes, the birth and a postnatal stay; at a Birth Centre you can have your baby and then go home. There are only two or three in the whole of the UK, so they may not be a realistic option for you. In 1999, expect prices to be in the region of £4–5k.

Pools and low tech care are available, but, as with other small units, transfer will be necessary if there is a problem. Both types guarantee continuity of care and one-to-one support in labour with a known midwife.

Private hospitals

If you are paying for your care, then you may find a local private hospital which caters for obstetric cases. These are rather thin on the ground, and most are in or near very big cities, or wealthy areas. They tend to be obstetrically dominated, but may have provision for midwife-led care.

ECR

If you have particularly strong, or clinical, reasons for requiring a system of care which is not available on the NHS, you may be able to arrange to have what is known as an Extra-Contractual Referral (ECR). This may apply if, for example, you have had a bad experience before, or are, perhaps, unable to get the care you want any other way. Write to the Director of Primary Care at your local Health Commission to plead your case and talk to your GP about the best way to obtain such a referral. The Association for Improvement in Maternity Services will be happy to advise you as well. Although it is theoretically possible to arrange an ECR yourself, most Commissions will expect your GP to write in support of your application and, even then, may not be in a financial position to grant your request, so don't hold your breath!

Making up your mind

You should be aware that where you choose to have your baby can affect the system of care you receive. If you choose a home birth, for example, you are more likely to get your antenatal visits at home and to have continuity of midwife in labour (although this is by no means certain). If you intend to organise your care to suit you, and would like some home visits, then talk to your community midwife about how this can be arranged. If there are difficulties over this, you could appeal to the Head of Midwifery to see if there is a way forward. If you work, then you are entitled to time off for antenatal visits and classes, but some people prefer to have evening or weekend appointments. You may be able to arrange this, but if it is that important, it is more likely that you will end up booking an independent midwife who will be able to see you at times which suit you, rather than the other way round!

Most maternity units have a list of factors, or booking criteria, which they consider might make the pregnancy more complicated:

1. Previous babies

5 or more
multiple pregnancy

2. Build

less than 5' tall
clinically obese

3. Previous medical history

diabetes
cardiac disease
renal disease or transplantation
deep vein thrombosis (a blood clot in a vein in the leg)
clotting disorders
haemoglobinopathies (blood diseases, such as thalassaemia)
pulmonary embolism (a blood clot on the lung)
epilepsy (fits)

4. Previous obstetric history

Caesarean section or hysterotomy (any surgical opening of the uterus)
proven cephalo-pelvic disproportion (where the baby is too big to fit through your pelvis)
rhesus antibody positive
previous stillbirth or neonatal death (not always)

5. Previous gynaecological history

pelvic floor repair
myomectomy (removal of fibroids)

6. Social status

current alcohol abuser
current substance abuser

These lists are often reviewed and items such as the height of the woman, or her weight, may be revised, and may not be considered to be an issue. You may not consider a particular item to be important in your case and make a decision based on what you feel to be best for you and your baby.

Broadly speaking, there are certain basic principles of care which are present everywhere:

- care shared between obstetrician, GP and midwife
- care given by GP and midwife
- care given by midwife only
- care given by an obstetrician.

You will probably want to see somebody early in your pregnancy and most women make the assumption that it has to be their GP. This is not necessarily so; you may prefer to see a midwife – all you need to do is make the appointment, either at the Health Centre or directly through the Head of Midwifery Services, who can be found at the local maternity unit. Although midwives share premises with GPs, they are not employed by them and are at liberty to see women in their own right.

Antenatal care exists to monitor your, and your baby's wellbeing. It isn't compulsory and you don't have to see anyone if you don't want to. You can choose which system of care you would like to receive and which best suits your needs. If those needs change at any point, you can discuss the options and review your choices, but ultimately, it's up to you. Very few women decide not to have antenatal care, as most feel reassured by having professional input and the research shows that pregnancy outcomes are better, but there are some who decide to go it alone.

If you send a midwife away because you don't like her, or what she's doing, you can ask the Head of Midwifery Services to provide a substitute, who you may find acceptable. In labour, if you decide not to have a midwife (or, indeed, any professional) in attendance, you should know that, if a midwife or doctor should turn up, only you can send them away. If anyone does this for you, they can be prosecuted for not permitting a midwife access to you.

In some areas, all women are referred to a consultant obstetrician unless they prefer not to see him or her. In this case, members of the obstetric team (senior registrar, registrar and senior house officer), may well only see you once, in the early part of the pregnancy, and again if the pregnancy continues beyond the due date. If your pregnancy is complicated by a factor such as diabetes, twins or high blood pressure, you will be advised to see more of the obstetric team than your GP and community midwife.

In other areas, just the GP and midwife care for women during pregnancy and, if you have decided to give birth in a hospital, you will be under the care of the hospital or community midwives for the birth and postnatal care. At any point in the pregnancy, the midwife or GP may refer you to an obstetrician if a specialist opinion is required. This system affords many advantages: you receive your care near to your home, avoiding travelling up to the maternity unit, and only women requiring specialist help are seen in the hospital, thus freeing up the time of the obstetrician and allowing sensible consulting times.

In areas where there are GP units with birthing and postnatal care facilities, the care given by the GP and midwife may be extended to birth care, too. The community midwifery service is usually organised around GP surgeries. Midwives are 'attached' to the surgery and work exclusively with those doctors, or, in the case of a small practice, with more than one practice. In some areas, the midwife and GP hold joint clinics; in others, they hold separate clinics with women visiting them alternately.

In the early days of antenatal care, a schedule was developed which suggested that women should be seen four-weekly from the initial visit until they were 28 weeks pregnant, then fortnightly from 28 to 36 weeks of pregnancy, and then weekly until they gave birth. This is, on average, 13 antenatal visits. Because pregnancy outcomes improved so dramatically when antenatal care was introduced, there has been a reluctance to change this pattern of visits. Research is currently underway to investigate the frequency and content of antenatal visits, to attempt to assess exactly what aspect of antenatal care is of the most value. Is it the number of visits, or what occurs during the consultation? Women themselves certainly value these visits and where new patterns have been tried out, there has been a measurable level of dissatisfaction, suggesting that the support and social aspects have to be added into the equation.

Current opinion suggests that women are seen too frequently and that nine or even five visits may be sufficient for those women having an uncomplicated pregnancy. Some places have already introduced these modified patterns of care, and you may find that your local unit is one of these.

The organisation of midwifery care in Trusts and Health Commissions is changing rapidly following the publication of *Changing Childbirth*. Many areas are already responding to the needs of women by initiating forms of care that provide more continuity of care. There is now a multitude of forms of midwifery care available across the country and there are more initiatives for midwives to care for women in their labour, as well as antenatally and postnatally. If continuity of midwife is very important to you, particularly at the birth, you should ask whether this will happen. Some women have reported instances in which they were promised continuity of care initially, but later in pregnancy, it became apparent that this would not be forthcoming. Remember that if promises fail to materialise, you can change your system of care at any point.

It is entirely possible for a woman to receive all her care from a midwife. As explained in Chapter 1, a midwife has a legal right to provide total care for a woman undergoing a normal pregnancy. This applies to all midwives, whether they work within the NHS or independently, and allows for greater continuity. Many women appreciate the specialist skills and advice of the midwife in pregnancy care.

If you rarely need to visit your GP, or have recently moved, the routine of antenatal visits provides an opportunity to meet and get to know your GP for the first time. There may well be times when you have to visit your GP with the baby and, if you have built up a relationship with him or her during the pregnancy, this will be helpful at these times. It is really up to you to decide for yourself who you find is most appropriate during your pregnancy and it is important that you know that you do, in fact, have a choice.

Care at the time of birth

The many new initiatives in team and group working mean that there is no standard form of care in labour. In those areas where conventional care is still practised, most women who have chosen to give birth in a hospital will be cared for by a hospital midwife who is based on the labour ward. They work in a shift pattern, providing a 24 hour service, usually in three shifts. These midwives become very skilled in the care of women in labour, in dealing with emergency situations and particularly with those women requiring intervention. They also become very skilled at forging relationships swiftly with women and their partners, and many midwives extend their shifts to complete the care of a woman.

In some areas there is provision for the community midwife to be involved with your labour. This very much depends on the level of support that is there to back up this midwife, for if she also has to provide all the antenatal and postnatal care for the women on her caseload, she may not be available to care for a woman in labour. Many midwives try to juggle their commitments (and lose a night's sleep!) to achieve this care in labour, and very often it is not them, but the system within which they work, which militates against this flexibility.

Independent midwives can and do give care in hospitals, although the vast majority consider homebirth as their field of expertise. The advantage of having a known midwife, however, is the preference of most of their clients.

Postnatal care

Women giving birth at home will receive all their care at home, unless a complication indicates a referral to a hospital, e.g. jaundice in the baby which requires treatment. Women who give birth in hospital may elect to go home directly from the labour ward, or to stay for a few days in a postnatal ward. Many women opt to go home after one night in hospital. This allows them to rest after the birth, and then go home to their familiar surroundings. There should, however, be someone to give them help and support at this time, as they recover physically from the exertion of childbirth, adapt to caring for their baby, and learn to cope with everyday living with a new baby.

Many hospitals have had to impose a limit on the length of stay that they may offer a woman after the birth of her baby, if the birth has been uncomplicated. In many units this is 48 hours, or two nights. This may be reduced in some hospitals, as smaller hospitals are closed and beds are at a premium in the remaining ones. In fact, there is evidence that a shorter stay in hospital reduces the incidence of infection of mothers and babies. If there is a complication or a problem, then naturally you would be encouraged to stay longer, or to spend a few days at your local community hospital, which may have postnatal beds.

Once at home you will be visited by your community midwife. This used to be a rigid daily visit until the 10th day when midwives would suddenly stop visiting. This is becoming much more flexible with midwives arranging with the mother how often and when they will visit, and for how long. Midwives have a legal responsibility until the baby is 28 days old, and the visits may be extended until the 28th day as needs determine. The visits are to offer support and advice about care and feeding, and to ensure that mother and baby are physically and emotionally well.

In short, there are enough systems of care for you to be able to find a service which meets your needs. Do be firm, and don't compromise your own well being. After all, you won't get another chance at having this baby, so the experience should be as good as you can make it.

1 These should be available from your midwife. If not, contact MIDIRS on 0800 581009 for details.

4

Antenatal preparation

Antenatal care is a comparatively recent innovation, which has developed in line with the increase in knowledge about the way in which pregnancies and babies progress. Certainly, with the advent of more and more screening tests, it has become possible to assess more accurately the condition of mothers and their babies. So much so, in fact, that the whole system of antenatal care is currently being reviewed in order to provide mothers with the level of care appropriate to their needs, rather than every mother having care, tests and visits which may not be necessary.

Some women may be offered more consultations than others if their pregnancy is troubled – for example, a woman with a previous history of repeated miscarriages may have more early visits so that any possible risks to the baby can be picked up. A woman who has had pregnancy-induced hypertension (also called pre-eclampsia – see below) may have more later visits in a subsequent pregnancy to check her blood pressure.

Early days

Many women find out they are pregnant one or two days after a missed period; this again is a recent development. Only in the last ten years have home tests been readily available which can detect a pregnancy as early as this, and it can have its disadvantages. For example, once you know you are pregnant, the next step is to go and see your midwife or doctor. Many women then feel very let down when all that happens is that they are told to come back when they are twelve or fourteen weeks pregnant. This is because most miscarriages happen in the first three months and, since these happen for a multitude of reasons, most of which can neither be foreseen nor prevented, it is customary for a woman to formally 'book' for her antenatal care at the end of the first three months. However, this varies from midwife to midwife and from doctor to doctor, and there are some who will offer at least one or two visits during these early days, mostly for support and encouragement. If you are badly affected by nausea, ask your midwife for advice – don't just put up with it in silence. There are lots of things you can try, ranging from ginger to sea bands, so do ask.

When you first discover you are pregnant, you should also be given some advice on taking folic acid. Ideally, you should start taking supplements of this vitamin about three months before conceiving. It helps to prevent spina bifida and if you haven't taken it before getting pregnant, you should certainly start now. If your GP won't prescribe it for you, you can buy it at your local chemist and they will advise you about the right dosage.

It is also important to make early contact if you think you may want to have a screening test such as Chorionic Villus Sampling (see below), as this should be done around the 10th week of pregnancy, or an early amniocentesis at about 12–14 weeks. You will need to be referred to an obstetrician for these tests and you should also be counselled about them, so make sure you visit your GP early if this is likely to be the case.

The first 'booking' appointment

You should be prepared for your first booking visit, whoever it is with, to take about an hour. By attending the booking visit, you are implicitly giving your consent to each procedure (blood pressure, urine testing and so on) so if you have any qualms, or uncertainties, about the procedures or processes, you should ask yourself whether it might not be better to have a discussion with the midwife first. If you have a phobia about needles, for example, it will be helpful for you to tell your doctor and midwife, as blood tests are recommended at intervals during pregnancy.

- You will be asked for the date of your last period, which will provide the basis for calculating when your baby is due. Do remember there are no guarantees – the average first pregnancy lasts 41 weeks and 1 day, and subsequent pregnancies 40 weeks and five days, so don't take your given date as gospel.

- You will be asked about your medical history, for example, whether you have had any heart or kidney disease, or whether you have needed treatment to achieve your pregnancy.

- You will be asked whether there is anything in your, or your partner's, family which may affect you or your baby, and about any previous pregnancies.

If you have information which you would prefer was kept confidential – a previous abortion, for example – then you should discuss this area of privacy thoroughly with the midwife at booking. If there are private areas of concern, then it's probably better to make an appointment at the Health Centre, on your own, before booking.

Your blood pressure will be checked, and this will be done on each visit. A rise in blood pressure later in pregnancy may indicate that you are at risk of developing pregnancy-induced hypertension (PIH, or pre-eclampsia), so it is useful to have a record of your blood pressure at this early stage.

You will have been asked to provide a urine sample which the midwife will test for protein and/or glucose. Another symptom of PIH is protein in the urine; your urine may also have protein if you have a urinary tract infection, so this is a useful way of diagnosing such disorders. Glucose is not normally present so, if a woman starts showing glucose in her urine, it may be a symptom of the sort of diabetes which can occasionally happen during pregnancy. The third symptom of PIH is water retention in the tissues of the body, known as oedema. Almost all women have some degree of oedema, particularly in their feet, legs and fingers, which is associated with a healthy pregnancy, but in PIH this is extended to include swelling of some internal tissues as well. See Chapter 7 for further details about this.

Finally, the midwife will examine your abdomen, to determine how much your uterus has grown. She may be able to hear the baby's heart at this early stage with a hand held heart monitor, but it may not be possible until a few weeks later.

Most midwives and doctors have stopped routinely weighing women now as it is not particularly useful. The research suggests that setting limits on weight gain makes no difference to the outcome of the pregnancy, and that all women should be treated as individuals in the matter of weight gained during pregnancy. There is every reason to eat a good mixed diet; it has been suggested that the essential fatty acids present in full cream milk and butter are valuable to a growing baby, so many women abandon the idea of 'low fat' while they are pregnant and eat natural foods.

At sixteen weeks you will be offered the opportunity to have various blood tests. These are

- to assess your iron levels in case you're anaemic (which may be offered again at 28 and 36 weeks)

- to find out your blood group and rhesus factor (rhesus incompatibility can have catastrophic effects on the baby – see Chapter 7)

- to carry out a test for blood antibodies (again, in case they affect the baby)

- to carry out a test for syphilis (undiagnosed, this can cause physical and mental disabilities in the baby)

• to carry out the Alphafetoprotein test (see below).

In some areas, you may be offered the Triple test (see below), and in a few (currently) a test for HIV antibodies. The last in particular should never be done without your express permission, or without counselling which answers all your questions and addresses any anxieties you may have.

You may accept or refuse any of these tests. Nobody can do tests, blood or otherwise, without your consent. You should be advised on the advantages (or not) of each one, and have the opportunity to discuss any potential consequences.

Subsequent visits will always involve the same checks – blood pressure, urine and any oedema will be noted. You will be asked about the baby's movements (these are usually first noticed from about 18 weeks with a first baby and from a couple of weeks earlier with second and subsequent babies) and the rate of the baby's growth will be measured. This is your opportunity to ask questions and discuss your wishes for the birth. If you are not going to have a midwife you know at the birth, it may be a good idea to write a birth plan so that whoever is there for the birth knows what is important to you.

Birth plans

Many Trusts incorporate a birth plan into their notes. These may be brief, simply asking whether you have any preferences in labour, or they may be quite detailed. A birth plan is only ever a set of guidelines, but these are your personal wishes. Events in childbirth are subject to change without notice, so expecting your birth plan to have the moral weight of the ten commandments is unrealistic. It is a very useful exercise, however, for you and, perhaps your partner, to talk together and write down the issues which matter to you. This way you make your needs quite clear and there is room for negotiation without compulsion.

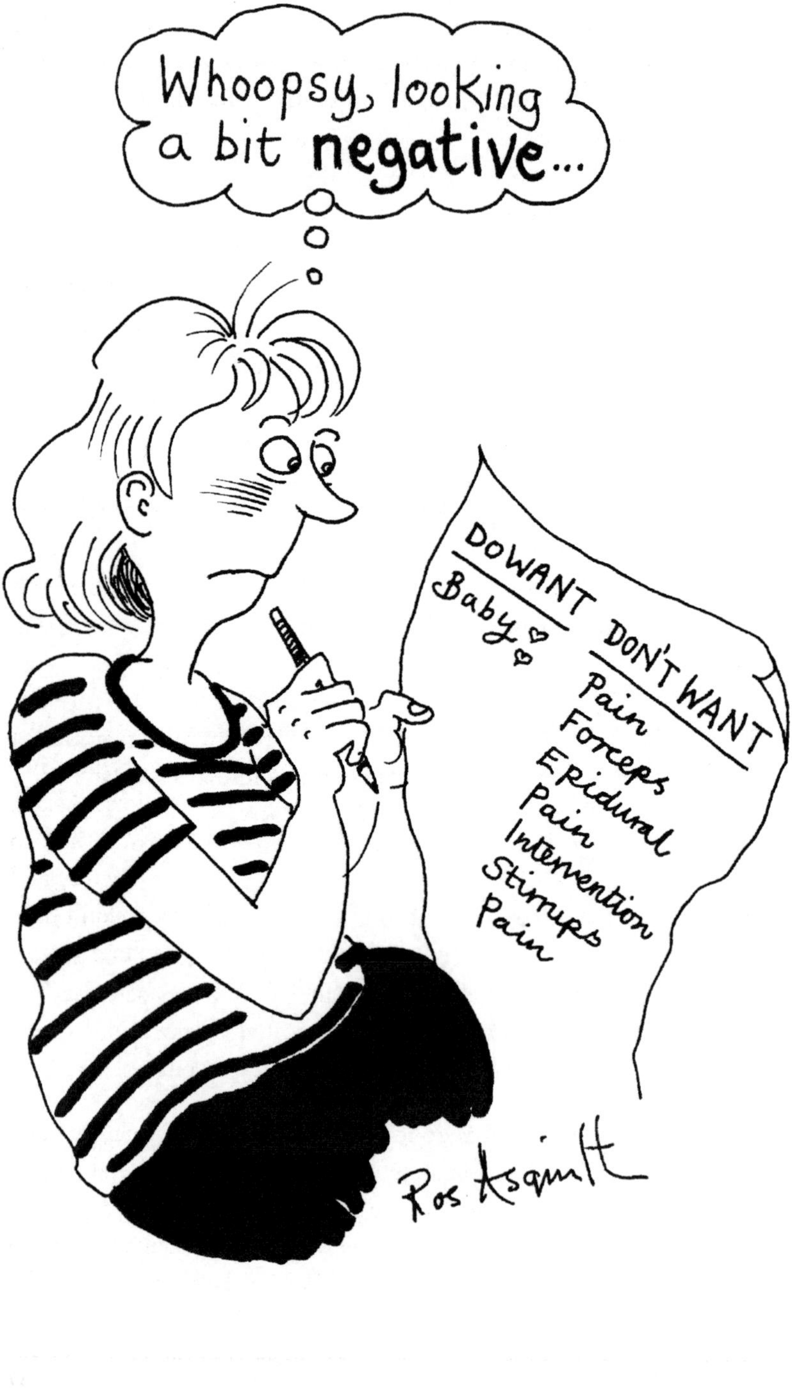

Whoopsy, looking a bit negative...
DO WANT
Baby
DON'T WANT
Pain
Forceps
Epidural
Pain
Intervention
Stirrups
Pain
Ros Asquith

Ideally, you would see the same people throughout your pregnancy, and discuss each subject with them, which would do away with the need for a plan, but more often continuity of carer is sadly lacking and a plan will give those who are, eventually, responsible for your care at the birth, a good idea of what is important to you.

The midwife will also advise you about your Social Security benefits, and at 28 weeks will give you a certificate which will enable you to get your maternity payments, if they are due to you. You should be given a booklet about these benefits, but if not you can pick one up at any post office.

Screening tests

Screening tests of various types are on offer throughout pregnancy, from very early ultrasounds through to fetal heart monitoring in labour. It is not the role of this book to recommend advisability or not − that's up to you − but it is important that you know to what you are agreeing.

Screening tests are not designed 'to make sure everything is all right', they are designed to see what, if anything, is wrong. If you would not contemplate having an abortion if you are carrying an abnormal baby, would you be better not having the test? Always take the time to discuss the implications fully with your midwife or doctor, and anybody else whose opinion is important to you. You shouldn't have any tests done which are not explained to you, and whose conse-quences, if any, you have not been warned about.

Chorionic villus sampling (CVS)

CVS or placental biopsy is done at 10–13 weeks of pregnancy and provides early detection of inherited disorders. For placental biopsy, a small sample of placental tissue is obtained either by a process similar to amniocentesis or by passing a fine tube through the vagina and cervix under ultrasound guidance. CVS involves passing a needle, usually through the mother's abdomen, into the amniotic fluid surrounding the baby and is associated with a small, but significant risk of miscarriage. The test may be offered to older women and those at risk of having a baby with certain inherited diseases. It is not 100% reliable, will not detect spina bifida and carries a 1–2% risk of miscarriage (higher than amniocentesis), so this should be discussed before undergoing the test. If CVS is appropriate for you, you may find it helpful to ask what the miscarriage rate following CVS is at your local centre, and compare it with a national centre, such as the one at King's College Hospital, before deciding where to go and who should do it.

Nuchal translucency scan

This is a relatively new technique. It involves measuring, via ultrasound scan, the size of a sac of fluid, which is present at this gestation, at the back of the baby's neck. It is performed at 11–13 weeks of pregnancy and is designed to flag up the possibility of chromosomal abnormalities, such as Downs Syndrome.

Amniocentesis

This test can be carried out anywhere between 12 and 18 weeks of pregnancy and is usually only offered to women over 35, women with a family history of spina bifida, Downs syndrome, muscular dystrophy, haemophilia, or cystic fibrosis and women with an abnormal AFP level. The test carries a 0.5% risk of miscarriage (this may vary from place to place), and you should always be advised what the test involves. You should also be counselled about possible consequences, before you agree to, or refuse, it. The test involves taking a small amount of amniotic fluid from around the baby and examining the chromosomes in the cells to identify any abnormality. It is performed by an obstetrician, who will inject a little local anaesthetic into the skin of your abdomen, over the uterus. Then, with the aid of an ultrasound scan, so that he or she can see where the needle is going, a needle is slipped into an area in the uterus where there is a good amount of liquor, and some of the fluid is syphoned out using a syringe. This fluid is then sent to a specialist laboratory where some of the cells are grown and the chromosomes identified. The results are usually available in two to three weeks.

Alphafetoprotein (AFP) test

This blood test may be performed at 16 weeks to assess the level of AFP in the mother's blood. High levels are associated with twins and triplets as well as babies with spina bifida, whereas low levels may occur when the baby has Down's syndrome. As high or low results can often occur when there is nothing at all wrong with the baby, and this is only a screening test, any abnormal levels would warrant a repeat blood test and further investigations such as ultrasound scan and/or amniocentesis.

Triple test

This test is specifically designed to detect Downs syndrome. It involves measuring AFP, human chorionic gonadotrophin and oestrogen in the mother's blood. The test is carried out at 16 weeks and is available on request, although in some areas you may have to pay to have it done. The results are not always reliable, and in any case only give an indication of the probability of a particular woman having a Down's Syndrome child. Further tests (such as amniocentesis) are always required if a positive result is obtained, as there are a high proportion of false positives and false negatives with this test.

Ultrasound scan

Most hospitals routinely offer an ultrasound scan at 18–20 weeks to confirm dates and look for any problems with the baby. However you may choose to have an early scan if there is some uncertainty as to your dates, or if a multiple pregnancy is suspected. You should be aware, however, that just because nothing abnormal is detected on scan, there is no guarantee that there is no hidden genetic abnormality.

Antenatal classes

Antenatal education

As your pregnancy progresses, you may like to go to antenatal classes. These will give you a good grounding in how to deal with labour and also help and advice concerning the first few weeks of parenthood. You are entitled to time off work for all your appointments and classes.

Most health centres and hospitals run their own antenatal classes, but these can sometimes be large groups and you may find them intimidating when it comes to raising questions of particular relevance to you. Often, several different people will teach at the classes, such as the midwives, a Health Visitor, or a physiotherapist. Ask your midwife whether there are any evening sessions that your partner can attend with you, who leads the classes, and what information/exercise groups are on offer from the NHS. The classes do have the advantage of being local, however, so this is a good opportunity to meet other pregnant women in your area and to do some networking. The class members may well end up as best friends as your babies grow up together. You may also be able to meet other midwives in the team and to have a look round the labour ward.

The National Childbirth Trust

The National Childbirth Trust runs classes in just about every area of the country (book early – classes are deliberately kept small, and fill very quickly). These are usually in the evenings, and are for you and your chosen birth partner to attend. Birth partners, whether they are your man, your mother, or your best friend, often feel hazy about their role or about what to expect and it can be very helpful for them to attend a set of structured classes. In this way, they can learn what they can do to help you, for example, massage routines that you

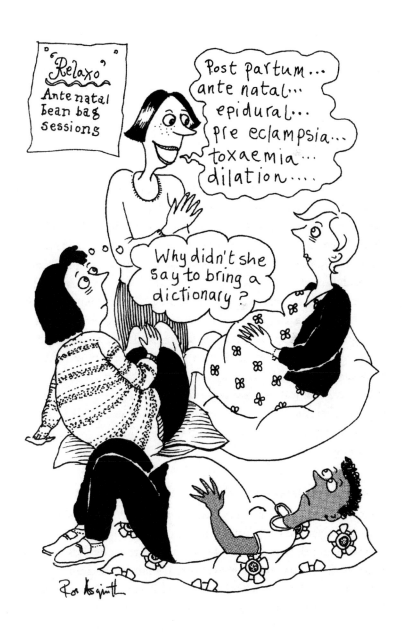

can practise together in advance. NCT teachers are mothers themselves, who have undergone a comprehensive training in order to become teachers. Each works with her local branch, looking after women in the area. The NCT also has breastfeeding counsellors, who will be available to you for help and advice during your pregnancy as well as afterwards. Once you have had the baby, you may find the NCT postnatal groups very helpful in those first months – or even years – as a new mother.

Active birth

Active Birth classes are for those who are planning to use exercise and movement in preparation for, and as part of, labour. These are not (yet) as widely available as the NCT, so if you want to attend these classes, you may have to be prepared to travel. They are usually for pregnant women only and are held during the day, but not always. You could also go to yoga classes, preparation for active birth, swimming (aquanatal) or stretch/tone classes. Most areas will have one or more of these classes especially designed for pregnant women, and this is a really good time to get fit. Aerobic exercise is not recommended during pregnancy, as the joints are too relaxed, but if you are accustomed to exercising regularly then you will probably want to find something which will maintain your fitness without putting a strain on the pregnancy. It is not a good time to begin strenuous exercise – if you do not usually take a lot of exercise, then start gently with yoga or swimming and work your way up to a level which feels comfortable and isn't a strain.

Exercise and exercise classes

Exercise in pregnancy is like exercise in general. It should be right for you, pitched at your level of fitness, fun and leave you with a feeling of well-being. Finding what is suitable for you depends on your lifestyle. The woman who cycles or attends aerobic sessions regularly will probably still cope with that for quite a way into her pregnancy. For those whose main form of exercise is walking to the car, however, heavy exercising in pregnancy is probably not such a good idea. Remember that whatever your fitness level, always listen to your body and aim to feel good, not exhausted!

Informal groups

In a few areas there are informal meeting groups. These are 'drop-in' sessions for women, with a midwife as a co-ordinator, where you can explore issues of interest or concern. Women often don't realise that they have a great deal of knowledge, and sharing this can be tremendously stimulating. Additionally, most areas have a homebirth support group, so if this is what you are planning, do get in contact with them.

Choosing a birth partner

This is the most incredibly important decision. The role of the birth supporter is not just to encourage, motivate and sustain you, but also to act as your advocate – to be your voice and to state your needs when you are too busy to do it yourself. Many women ask their husbands or partners to perform this role for them, and many are proud and privileged to do so.

But what if your partner doesn't feel he or she can take on the responsibility? Perhaps they hate hospitals, are stricken speechless by the sight of bodily fluids, or would be unable to cope with your pain? What if they are in the services and will be thousands of miles away? The person you choose must be up to the job; if they are asked and feel unable to take it on, then both of you will feel bad – they will feel guilty and you will feel rejected.

Your birth supporter must be there for you. They are not there to make conversation with the professionals, or to persuade you to accept treatment you don't want, they are there to help you give birth to your baby and that is too important to leave until the last minute. If you are unable to have your life partner with you, for whatever reason, then draw up a short list. Look at friends and relations with an assessing eye. Talk to your midwife – is she somebody you'd like to have with you?

Approach the subject cautiously, talk about the general idea and see how it's received. Try to avoid people who will see themselves as somehow more important than any of your other friends and family because they've been Chosen; avoid those who seem likely to say yes to anything and then wimp out at the last minute. What you need is someone who cares about you and what happens to you; someone strong, who will take your side; someone to watch over you, who isn't afraid of the physical side and who will rise to the occasion with style and aplomb. You'll find them. They're out there, waiting for you to ask!

5

Labour

There seems to be a great deal more to pregnancy and labour than just having a baby. There are all sorts of discoveries to be made about yourself and your relationships. Many women find, for example, that they identify much more closely with their mothers after having their own baby, and see themselves as the latest link in a long chain going through the ancestral mists.

For those having their first babies, labour is wholly uncharted territory. At some point, you may ask a friend who has a child, "What does a contraction feel like?". You will then be quite irritated when she goes all vague and lost for words – it sounds as if she is being unnecessarily secretive. She isn't. There simply aren't the words to explain a contraction to anyone who has never had one, because the terms of reference simply aren't there and a contraction isn't like anything else. One day, a friend who is pregnant will ask you the same question and you'll hear yourself doing exactly the same – being vague and lost for words.

Most women seem to get to about the 28th week of their pregnancy and then suddenly realise that, no matter what happens now, the baby has to come out. This may sound self-evident, but there's nothing quite like that first, crashing realisation of the inevitability of it all. It's about this time that the tentative planning begins. We are all the sum of our experiences and bring to parenthood all the impressions, feelings and prejudices that make us what and who we are. It's

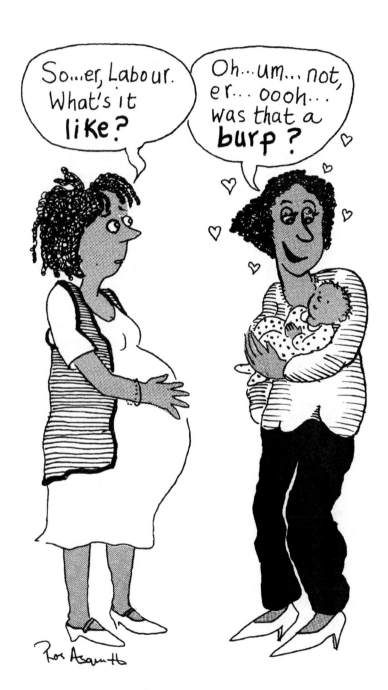

the same with labour. For some women, having the baby in hospital, with all the kit there, 'just in case', is of supreme importance. For others, the safety and security of home is what matters most. Some women find that pregnancy brings with it hitherto undisclosed fears; their stress levels and anxiety go sky high and they are unable to relax and enjoy what is happening. In these, and many other aspects, ignorance equals fear. Stories you may have half-heard as a child, lack of knowledge about how the body functions in labour, all these things go towards creating fear and mystery about something that is as basic (and as wonderful) as the sunrise.

In this chapter, I have tried to use the words that you will hear used by midwives and doctors when you go into labour, with explanations of their meaning. This way, I hope you won't feel excluded from discussions by the use of unfamiliar jargon.

First of all, then, what does the body do and how does the whole thing work? Normal labour is divided into three stages (but look out for the subdivisions!):

- First stage: the opening of the cervix from its normal, closed state, to fully open
- Second stage: the birth of the baby
- Third stage: the delivery of the placenta and membranes.

The purpose of labour is to open the cervix, in order to permit the exit of the baby from the uterus, down the vagina and into the outside world. This happens by means of muscular contractions, which start at the top of the uterus and pull upwards on the cervix. The uterus is a unique organ, in that each of these contractions leaves the muscle fibres microscopically shorter than before. The effect of this shortening is seen in the cervix as it is gradually drawn up (effaced) and opened (dilated).

At the same time, the baby moves down in the uterus and, consequently, in the pelvis, which acts as a protective framework. Although

Figure 5.1
Before labour starts

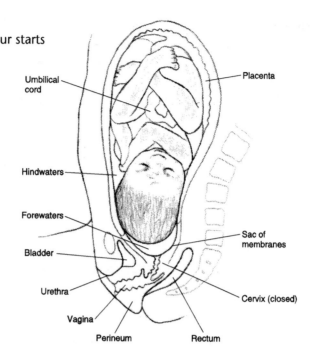

Umbilical cord

Placenta

Hindwaters

Forewaters

Bladder

Urethra

Vagina

Perineum

Rectum

Sac of membranes

Cervix (closed)

Figure 5.2
Start of active labour

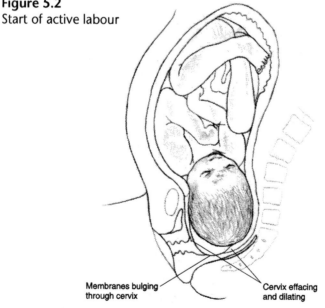

Membranes bulging through cervix

Cervix effacing and dilating

The baby is deeper into the pelvis and more curled up

Figure 5.3
End of first stage

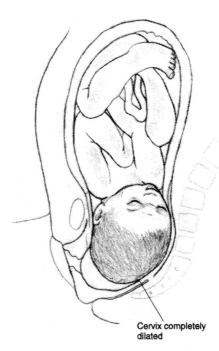

Cervix completely
dilated

Figure 5.4
Second stage – baby's
head crowning,
membranes have
ruptured

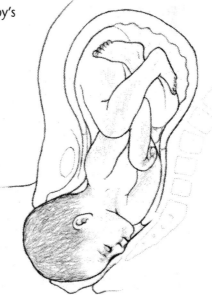

See how the angle of the head turns within the pelvis

Figure 5.5
Towards the end of
second stage – head
delivering

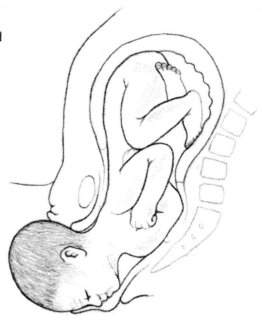

the mechanism by which labour starts is not certain, the process of labour is maintained through a circular release of hormones. These hormones are released through an interaction between mother and baby – in other words, everyone concerned is going to work very hard indeed!

The hormone which causes the uterus to contract is oxytocin. It is released by the mother's pituitary gland. The hormone which induces the pituitary to produce oxytocin is prostaglandin, which is released when the cervix is stimulated. Stimulation of the cervix occurs through pressure from the baby's head, the bulge of the membranes inside and the effect of contractions. This is the reason why upright labouring positions are so beneficial – they allow gravity to play its part by bringing the pressure from the head onto the cervix, thus increasing the degree of cervical stimulation (see Figure 5.2).

If this is your first baby, the thinning and shortening (effacement) will probably occur completely before your cervix begins to dilate.

Effacement (and up to 3–5cm dilation) is often referred to as the 'latent first stage', or 'pre-labour', and can take place over the last couple of weeks, or days, before labour becomes 'established', which is when the cervix has dilated to about 4–5 cm and the contractions are strong and regular.

During this time, you may experience the cardinal signs of labour:

- You may have a show

- Your membranes may rupture ('breaking the waters')

- You may have regular, painful contractions.

All three of these events may happen, or possibly only one (usually the contractions). You may notice other things, like wanting to clean the house from top to bottom, a sense of restlessness, or, conversely, wanting to lie quietly in a dark space. You may have frequent bowel movements. Any or all of this is completely normal and will vary from one pregnancy to another.

The show

In the early first stage of labour, as your cervix is beginning to thin, shorten and dilate, you may notice the plug of thick mucus which fills the cervical canal coming away. This is called a 'show' and when it happens, you will have a vaginal discharge of blood and mucus mixed together, which can sometimes be quite copious. If you are unsure, or are concerned that the discharge is blood, rather than blood and mucus, then contact your midwife or doctor for advice.

You need to know, however, that the show can occur up to two weeks before labour starts, so don't get too excited about it. Although women count a show as being significant, it really is only an indicator that the cervix is softening and ripening in readiness for labour, rather than a sign that labour is starting.

Rupture of the membranes

There are a few myths surrounding the waters breaking. You may hear women say that an early rupture of the membranes leads to 'a dry labour'. This is not so – there's no such thing. As long as the membranes remain in the uterus, the water surrounding the baby (liquor) continues to be made. You may also be told that early breaking of the waters means a long hard labour. There is no research evidence to support this either.

As a general rule, the membranes do not break until your cervix is 8–10 cm dilated, when the pressure inside the uterus reaches a critical point. In some cases, however, particularly if the baby's position is occipito-posterior (his back to your back), they may break early, even before the cervix has begun to dilate. When your waters break, you should let your midwife know. She may want to check that all is well by examining you and listening to the baby's heartbeat.

When the sac (bag) of membranes surrounding the baby breaks, liquor is released. In some cases, this will be a slow trickle; it may be that the baby's head is well down in the pelvis and acting like a cork, or it may be what is called a 'hindwater rupture'. This occurs when the membranes break higher in the uterus, releasing liquor from above the 'presenting part' (usually the baby's head, or bottom, if it's breech). If the head is not fully 'engaged' (that is, if it is higher in the pelvis), then there may well be a flood – and no doubt whatsoever that the waters have gone.

If the presenting part is well down, there may be some doubt as to whether the membranes have broken. If they have, then the trickle will persist – try putting a sanitary pad on; if, after an hour, the pad is wet, then it's almost certainly liquor. The trouble is that many women get caught out when the baby does a sudden handspring on your bladder, causing a leak of urine. If it is that, then unless you have severe incontinence problems, all you will get is a quick leak and the pad will be dry after an hour.

You should look at the colour of the liquor. It should be clear, or straw-coloured and may have white flecks of vernix (the thick, creamy substance that covers the baby's skin while it's in the uterus) in it. If the liquor is greenish, or brown in colour, the baby may have passed meconium, the first bowel movement. It's thick, sticky and dark greenish-brown in colour, a cross between tar and porridge! This may well influence professional opinions on how your labour should be managed. There are two causes for meconium being present in the liquor: one is that if babies are distressed for some reason, the anal sphincter relaxes and the stool is passed. The other is that a stool may be passed, simply because the baby's bowel is full. For a discussion on the management of meconium stained liquor, see Chapter 7.

Contractions

It is this latent phase which leads women to consider that they have been in labour for days, whereas, in fact, the active, or established, phase of labour only lasts a few hours. It can be devastating to discover, after you've been contracting all night, that your cervix is barely dilated. It is for this reason that most midwives and antenatal teachers will tell you to ignore these early contractions as much as possible, and to realise that they are probably only readying the cervix for labour, rather than actually labouring. It is also important to know that your contractions may feel intense, but not consistent in length, strength, or frequency. This is quite normal for this stage.

Conserving your energy and pacing yourself is very important. Often when contractions first begin there is much excitement because, after all, you've been waiting for this baby for some time. At this stage in the proceedings, try to ignore what's happening and just live your life. You won't miss anything, I promise! If it's night time and you start contracting, then take two paracetamol, have a warm bath and go to bed. The best thing you can do, especially at night, is to rest and try to sleep. There is no advantage in walking about to try to keep the contractions going; all that happens is that you get exhausted and the contractions will still come or go, according to their own rhythm.

Try to temper your excitement. You may want your partner with you at this stage, but it is important that you realise that the latent phase of the first stage may last for 24 hours or more, and anxiety or stress may well prolong this time. Continue as much of your normal day to day activity as you can. Try going for a walk round the block, or in the park, at your leisure, but remind yourself periodically to relax mentally and physically.

You need to be able to labour in an anxiety-free frame of mind. This is a good time to get the baby-sitters in if you have another child, so that you aren't concerned about their well-being. All these arrangements should be made well in advance, along with packing the bags and stocking the freezer.

When the contractions begin to get painful, try getting in a deep warm bath. This will either slow the contractions, or move the labour into the active stage. The contractions will not ease or stop if your body is ready for strong/active labour, but warm water will help you to relax. Water is a great relaxant and an excellent form of pain relief especially if you can use a pool which gives you the opportunity to submerge. Sitting on a (plastic!) chair in the shower with the water spraying onto your back may also provide you with relief.

Do make sure that if you want to eat and drink, you do. You may not feel very hungry, so stick to high energy, easily digestible foods, such as scrambled egg, pasta or cereals. Drinks can include anything you feel able to tolerate – sweet fizzy drinks, milk, or clear soup are good examples, as they also contain 'easy access' calories. When you are in labour, once you have used up all your accessible energy stores, you start burning muscle tissue. This gives rise to a situation akin to starvation – your breath will smell of acetone, and there will be a measurable level of ketones in your urine – and your contractions may well slow down and become ineffectual. So, eat, or don't eat, according to what your body tells you.

It's worth noting that your position can help or hinder the process. If you're upright, not only do you have the advantage of gravity, but also an improved blood flow to the uterus. When muscles are starved of oxygen, they will not work as efficiently as they might, and contractions will be more painful, so keeping mobile and upright is a good start (see Figures 6.1 and 6.2).

Is this it?

The normality of labour is predicated upon whether progress is being made. This progress is measured by the rate and degree of cervical dilatation, and the descent through the pelvis of the 'presenting part' (the head, if the baby is in a cephalic position, the bottom if it's breech).

How far down into the pelvis the baby has gone can be assessed by palpating your abdomen, but the only sure way to tell if your cervix is dilating is to have a vaginal examination (VE). The midwife wears sterile gloves and will gently insert two fingers into your vagina, using a lubricant gel, so that she can estimate the degree of effacement and dilatation of the cervix. There is always a risk that VEs can introduce infection, particularly if your membranes have ruptured, so these are kept to a minimum.

It is also possible to check the baby's position, and how far down in the pelvis he is. This check is usually done at each VE, as the further along in labour you are, the lower the baby; it's a mark of progress. The more relaxed and accepting of the procedure you are, the easier and quicker it is.

Some women may find the idea of an internal examination repugnant, for a variety of reasons – in particular, women who have been abused or assaulted. Nobody can examine you without your permission, of course, so the control is in your hands. If this is difficult for you, talk to your midwife or doctor and explain how you feel. Discussing it in advance gives people time to consider options. Some women find that talking their worries over with a counsellor is very useful.

If you have been abused or assaulted, it may be difficult for you to say so, particularly at this point, so it is important for you to tell somebody, in some way, during your pregnancy. If you are not able to tell your midwife or GP, perhaps your partner, or a relative or close friend, could do it for you. If that isn't possible, then Rape Crisis Counsellors can be extraordinarily helpful, but the earlier in your pregnancy you seek help, the better.

Making contact

So, there you are, contracting away – when do you let your midwife or the hospital know? There are many components to this equation, so consider the following (preferably in advance) and discuss them with your midwife and your labour partner:

- If you are not having your baby at home, how far away from the hospital do you live?

- How long will it take you to get there? Residents of large cities need to consider the effects of rush hour, as well.

- Is it possible to arrange for your community midwife to come and assess you when you think you are in labour, to save you a possibly wasted journey?

- If this is not your first baby, how long did you labour last time? Second babies tend to arrive much faster and labour establishes itself more quickly.

- If this is your first baby, is there a family history of quick labours?

- Do you have somebody to be with you while you are in labour? If not, how are you going to get to the place where you plan to have your baby?

- Have you been advised to go to hospital sooner rather than later for any reason – for example, twins, or a low lying placenta?

Once you think you are in labour – the 'This Is It' frame of mind – consider the following:

- Have you been told to contact someone as soon as you think things are starting?

- Are you confident to carry on, or are you looking for some reassurance?

- How long have you been at it – are you exhausted?

- Are you on your own?

- Have your waters broken?

If the answer to any of these is 'yes', then you would be well advised to contact your midwife, or the hospital, for advice and guidance. Contented, settled women will labour more efficiently than tense, anxious ones, so I should also add that the decision of when to make contact is up to you; you may choose to phone when you have your first contraction, or not until you feel that you need someone professional with you. Take into account whether your pregnancy has been normal, how you feel in yourself and do what seems to be the right thing for your baby and for you.

Knowing when you are in established labour can be tricky. After all, it is an empirical judgment, based on an assessment of cervical progress, and the length, strength and closeness of contractions. Some women can get to eight centimetres dilated on very few contractions, others will contract every two minutes, for a long time, to get there. You may ask whether it is, really, important to know? When there are so many variables in the limits of normal labour, is it appropriate to expect women to follow a pattern imposed upon them?

Active management of labour

Some hospitals use a system of care known as 'active management of labour', which is based upon the premise that no woman should be in labour for longer than twelve hours, but this programme is not based upon individualised care. It is based upon research done in Ireland, which used a combination of procedures, such as accurate diagnosis of the onset of labour; rupturing the membranes; the use of drugs to stimulate the uterus and a midwife who stayed with the woman throughout. For some women, the time limit is ideal, but for others, the level of intrusive procedures seems unacceptably high.

Where this programme has been implemented in the UK, however, the midwifery element has been left out and the outcomes do not equate to the Irish ones. In particular, increased numbers of women have had Caesarean sections and many have expressed dissatisfaction with this form of care. You could assume from this that the continuous presence of a known midwife is of significant importance in achieving outcomes which are as good psychologically as they are physically. If your local hospital practises active management, you may find it useful to talk to your midwife in order to find out exactly what is involved and what your options are.

Established labour

Once you are in established labour, you may find it very difficult to focus on anything that is going on except what's happening to you. Your sense of time becomes distorted – five minutes can seem like two hours and vice versa. You may need all your energy to deal with the contractions, and communication is reduced to the bare necessities; saying 'please' and 'thank you' simply takes too much time!

This is the time when your birth partner is so important. You may want your back rubbed, or the TENS electrodes moved, or a cold flannel for your face, or just someone to cling to – particularly if you don't have your own midwife with you. Your partner is the one who reminds you to empty your bladder at regular intervals (every couple of hours or less), gives you drinks, holds the bag of sweets, gets the ice chips, knows where the sandwiches are. All these things are so small and so important. Your partner's hand is the one that gets crushed. Your partner is the one who hugs you and tells you you're wonderful and so clever, when you feel as if it's all getting too much. It's a crucial role. Every home should have one.

Some midwives do very few internal exams, knowing that they can usually tell how a woman is getting on by the way she moves, looks and sounds, how long the contractions last, how strong they are and how often they are coming. It takes a great deal of experience and confidence for midwives to work in this way, and in most hospitals, midwives are expected to make a formal assessment every four hours or so when you are in normal, active labour.

Prolonged labour can, however, exhaust mother and baby, which may lead to fetal distress. It may also be a sign that there is something wrong with the process, so it is important that your progress in active labour is assessed, especially if it seems to be going on for a very long time. You may want to know what is going on, too, so that you can pace yourself or ask for pain relief if you want it.

Transition

This is the awkward time between first and second stages of labour, with the cervix from about 8–10cm dilated. The contractions are incredibly strong; often you will just not know what to do with your-self – even your skin doesn't seem to fit properly. Nobody can do any-thing right and you just want the whole thing over and done with. It hurts. It is often at this point that women ask for pain relief, feeling that they just can't carry on. You may become tearful and demoralised, unable to see any relief or ending, and totally forgetting why you're in this state at all, so it is extremely helpful if somebody reminds you that this is transition and you're nearly there. Being aware of what is happening to you is half the battle, so your partner should remind you about the breathing patterns you've practised in your antenatal classes, breathing with you to help you with the rhythm.

You will need help at this stage to change your position. Your partner can help you to get upright. Everyone feels better and stronger if their head is higher than the pain, so kneeling up, or leaning over pillows will be helpful. Even if you're being monitored, you can still get into a position which enables you to work with the forces inside you.

That said, not everybody notices a transitional period. They contract away and then suddenly hear a grunting noise, which, they realise in astonishment, came from their own throat. To your amazement, you've done it, after all. You're ready to have a baby!

6

Pain relief

At some point during your pregnancy you will have to consider whether you are likely to want to use pain relief in labour and, if so, to weigh up the benefits and disadvantages of each option available. Pain relief comprises whatever helps you to cope with your labour. You are the only one who can decide what is best for you, but you need to know what the side effects and ramifications of your choice are likely to be.

Exhaustion and hunger can increase your need for pain relief, as will giving birth to your baby in a place in which you do not feel comfortable, or in the company of strangers. The research shows that having someone you know with you during labour reduces the length of labour and the need for pain relief. This, ideally, would be your midwife, but it may be a birth companion – your partner, antenatal teacher, or a close friend – who gives you this essential support. You may choose to have a couple of people to act as birth companions, but discuss this with your midwife, as some hospitals put a limit on the number of people in a labour room. At home, of course, you can have as many people around you as you like.

It is important to realise that decisions which seemed right at the time may not seem right when you are actually in labour. If, for example, you decide in advance that you definitely don't want an epidural, but then in labour you need one, you may feel that in some way you have failed yourself. If you need pain relief, then take it – make expedient decisions at the time. Labour is a marathon, not

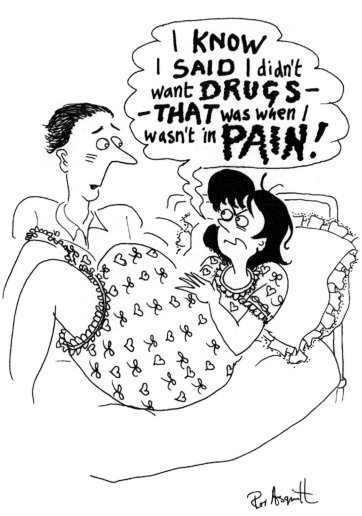

martyrdom. Just make sure you know what is likely to be involved and then you will be able to make an informed decision in the light of current circumstances.

You may find it useful to look at the birth stories at the back of the book, to see how other women coped.

Relaxation

Probably the most important thing is to accept that you are not in control of what is happening to you. You are not in a position to actually control the pain you feel, but you are in a position to control your response to it. Relax – 'fall forwards' into your contractions and

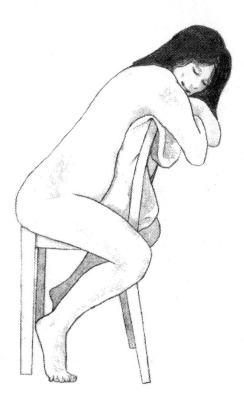

Figure 6.1 Comfortable sitting position for first stage of labour

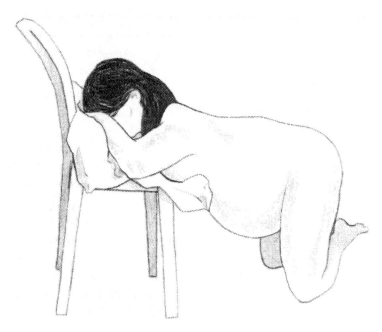

Figure 6.2 Comfortable kneeling position for first stage of labour

let them do their work. Being confident in your knowledge of what is happening will help a great deal, as fear often makes perceived pain a great deal worse by causing tension and physical stress. Relaxation is one of the most useful life skills you can learn.

Breathing patterns are very important, as they enable you to control the visible signs of stress which we all, to a greater or lesser degree, exhibit. Some of us are shoulder hunchers, some are teeth grinders, some clench their fists and so on. All these responses have the effect of tightening groups of muscles, which makes it difficult to relax. The trick is to learn to recognise these responses in yourself, and to treat their presence as a trigger response for relaxation. Once you have learned to control these external stress symptoms, your body will relax and encourage labour to progress.

It's no good learning to relax lying down comfortably – you need to learn relaxation as a skill, so that you can do it, (for example, while you're driving), with your eyes open! Yoga classes, active birth preparation, the NCT – all these teach practical, effective relaxation, as well as breathing skills for labour. The skills you learn will stand you in good stead for other areas of your life, which are likely to be stressful – such as parenting!

In the active/established phase your contractions will make you stop and work on your breathing rhythm; they are likely to be intense. However, you should also concentrate on relaxing between contractions and focus on conserving your energy. Go with your contractions; put your brain into neutral, don't fight them. You will find it easier, at this point, to surrender to forces outside your control. Move as your instincts tell you and remember to keep yourself as upright as possible. Many women are sick at some point in labour, and a few will be frequently sick – this is normal, it's just a physiological response, but it's best to be prepared for such eventualities.

Take all the support available – back massage, kind words, nice smells, good music – all these help to create an ambience of peace and relaxed calm, so that you can focus on the job in hand.

Epidural anaesthetic

An epidural is really a local anaesthetic. It is always administered by an anaesthetist who has had special training in this procedure with women in labour. A drip is put into one of the veins in your hand or arm and you will then be put into a position which enables you to curl up, so that your spine is well curved. The anaesthetist will insert a very fine, flexible plastic tube (a catheter), through a hollow needle which is put in at about waist level between the vertebrae. Local anaesthetic is used for the initial injection – you may feel some pressure in your back, but nothing else. Once the fine catheter is in place, local anaesthetic is injected through it – a test dose first – and, if there are no ill effects, the full dose is given. This will last a couple of hours or so and will then need to be topped up, or you may have a pump attached to the line which will give a continuous low dose flow. The procedure usually takes about twenty minutes, once the anaesthetist has arrived.

Your blood pressure will need to be monitored, as an epidural will cause it to drop (if you have high blood pressure in pregnancy, you may be advised to have an epidural for this very reason), so you may have a midwife in attendance in the room all the time, to check your condition. The baby will need to be on a monitor (a cardio-tocographic – CTG – trace) to check the heartbeat and its response to your contractions. With a mobile epidural, the baby's heartbeat will be recorded on a CTG while you are first given the anaesthetic, and subsequently during top-ups, but if all is well, then the midwife will listen in at intervals between these top-ups. If you need to have a Caesarean section, an epidural will ensure that you are awake and alert for the birth, and also that you will feel better more quickly than if you had a general anaesthetic.

Points to bear in mind:

- This is the only procedure which will give you total pain relief. Sometimes, however, there are places which are not affected and it can be distressing to feel concentrated sensation in one small spot. If you are having a great deal of back pain in labour, or you are exhausted, an epidural can feel like a life-saver.

- 20–30% of women have one (depending on the area); twice as many first timers as others. 75% said it gave very good total pain relief, 18% said it was good, 5% said it didn't help. (Source: National Birthday Trust)

- In most places, you will lose the use of your legs while the epidural is effective, and so you will have to stay on a bed.

- Some hospitals offer a mobile epidural which enables you to walk about, but because you can't feel anything in the pelvic area, you do need to be very careful how you move.

- You have to keep still during the procedure, which can be difficult when you are contracting strongly, so don't surrender control until you find you are pain-free. Entonox can be helpful at this point.

- The contractions may slow down, or even stop under the influence of the epidural, so you may need a hormone drip (which will be attached to the original one) to get them going again. Epidurals are associated with longer labours.

- You may not be able to push effectively, so you are more likely to need forceps or ventouse to help the baby out.

- You can only have an epidural where there are anaesthetists on 24 hour call, which rules out small GP units and homebirths. Also, if the anaesthetist is busy in theatre, for example, then you'll have to wait, which can be distressing.

- There is a chance (0.6–1.8%) that the needle may accidentally puncture a layer of the membrane surrounding the spinal cord, causing what is known as a dural tap. This will give you a nasty headache and may necessitate you having a forceps delivery. The effects generally last for 24–48 hours.

- Some women complain of backache following epidural. The Royal College of Anaesthetists recommends that women should have their backs well supported until the effects have worn off to prevent unfelt muscle or ligament strain occurring.

- You may have difficulty emptying your bladder under epidural. This will mean that the midwife will have to empty it for you, using a urinary catheter passed into the bladder to drain the urine.

Pethidine

This is a synthetic (man-made) opiate drug, which has a similar action to drugs such as morphine. It is given by injection into your thigh or buttock and takes about twenty minutes to start working. The standard dose is between 100–150 mg, but small women, or those in early labour, may benefit from a half or even a quarter dose. As pethidine routinely causes nausea and vomiting, it is given with an anti-emetic to prevent sickness. For some women the sedation is enough – it will relax them and take the edge off the contractions, especially if given early.

Points to bear in mind

- Pethidine is usually available wherever you choose to have your baby.

- About 40% of women use it. 25% said it was very good, 25% said it was no help. (Source: National Birthday Trust)

- Its effect is more of a sedative than an analgesic, which means that it will put you to sleep rather than curing the pain.

- It can slow down the contractions, making it necessary for them to be stimulated by an oxytocin drip. Alternatively, you may wake up to find yourself in full labour. This can be difficult to deal with, as you will have a tendency to drop off to sleep between contractions and wake just as the contraction reaches its peak. It is very difficult to get your breathing co-ordinated under these circumstances.

- It is a mood enhancer. This means that whatever you are feeling emotionally when you have the injection, may be exaggerated by it.

- Some women have hallucinations whilst under the influence of pethidine.

- You will feel drunk and your legs will be unsteady, so you will probably have to stay put after having the injection. Most hospitals will not let you use the pool if you have had pethidine.

- There is evidence to suggest that pethidine given at any time during labour will affect the baby. The baby will be sleepy and may be reluctant to feed for up to 72 hours, which can mean that you have difficulty in establishing breastfeeding.

- The optimum effect is reached about two hours after administration. If the baby is born at this point, the pethidine may depress his respiratory centre and he will not breathe properly. If this happens, he will be given an injection of naloxone, which is an antidote to pethidine.

Entonox (gas and air)

Entonox is a 50/50 mixture of nitrous oxide and oxygen, which is breathed in through a mask or mouthpiece, administered by the woman to herself. The effects are similar to being a bit drunk, but dissipate in less than a minute (and there's no hangover!), although you may still feel the effects for twenty minutes or so, after using entonox continuously. It will not cure the pain, but many women find it takes the edge off it, enabling them to cope.

The trick to using entonox is to remember that there is a time lag between breathing the gas in and when it starts to work, so you need to start inhaling it as soon as the contraction begins, rather than waiting until you can feel the pain. This ensures maximum effect at the height of the contraction. You should take big, deep breaths which fill your lungs (but be careful not to hyperventilate), which will not only fit in with, but also help you concentrate on, the breathing patterns that you have been taught. Many women feel it also helps by giving them 'something to do'.

If you are having a home birth, there is a possibility that the supply of entonox may be limited, as there are only so many cylinders that the midwife can fit in the boot of her car. If you use it all, further supplies will have to be brought, and this may mean a slight delay.

Points to bear in mind:

- Entonox is available everywhere – homebirths, ambulances, GP units and hospitals.
- About 75% of women use it, and 84% said it was good or very good. (Source: National Birthday Trust)

- You can use it in conjunction with any other form of pain relief, or for short periods, such as while you are waiting for an epidural, or while being stitched. You can also use it in a birth pool.

- It is self-administered, which has the advantage that if you over breathe it, all that happens is you drift off to sleep, your hand holding the apparatus falls away from your mouth and you start breathing normal air again.

- It is supplied via rubber tubing and a mask (if no mouthpiece is available) and some people find the smell of rubber nauseating.

- It can make some women feel sick and dizzy.

- It can be dehydrating to use for a long time (because you have to breathe through your mouth) so you should also make sure that you have plenty to drink and have sips of fluid, if possible, between every contraction.

- Many midwives suggest that women start using it towards the end of first stage, from about 7–8 cm dilated onwards, as it may not be as effective if used for long periods.

- You may be asked to stop using it in the second stage of labour, while pushing, as it helps if you are alert at this point!

TENS (transcutaneous electronic nerve stimulation)

Four battery operated electrodes are fastened onto your back, either with tape or self-adhesive. You should be shown where to put them to get the optimum effect (Figure 6.3). The apparatus is controlled by a 9v battery in a little box about the same size as a cigarette packet which can be clipped to a belt or put in your pocket. These electrodes pulse electrical stimulation at a rate which stimulates the production of the body's natural painkillers, endorphins. They also scramble messages from the nerves in that area, making it hard for the pain signals to get to the brain. As the contractions increase in length, strength and frequency, so you increase the length, strength and frequency of the electrical pulses. You should start using TENS as early as possible

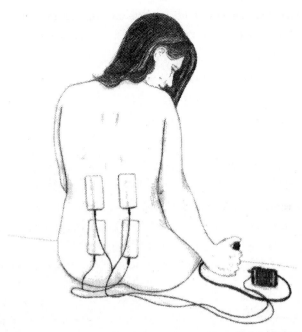

Figure 6.3 Transcutaneous electronic nerve stimulation (TENS)

in labour for the best effect and it may also be helpful if you try using it beforehand. It can help alleviate backache in late pregnancy, so this is a good opportunity to practise.

Points to bear in mind:

- It's under your own control and you can use it where and when you like, right from the beginning of labour.
- There have been no reported side effects on women or their babies.
- Research suggests it is more helpful in early labour, especially for first timers.
- You can't use it if you if you have a heart pacemaker or are labouring in water, but you can use it before you get into the pool.
- You can't have your back massaged if you're wearing a TENS machine.

- If your baby needs to have his heartbeat monitored electronically, you may be asked to remove your TENS.

- You will have to pay to hire one if your local midwife or hospital doesn't have one that you can borrow.

Water

The use of water as pain relief has been well known for centuries – it's called hydrotherapy and is used for rheumatic pain, as well as muscular aches and strains. Many women find a bath enormously relaxing and when you're in labour it's no different, except that complete immersion in the water, so that you float freely, is most important. Whilst water cannot provide complete pain relief, it can certainly make things more comfortable, as it acts as a support and helps in the production of endorphins. Water will make you feel more mobile and lighter, as well as soothing you mentally. Most women who choose to labour in water do so in specially designed pools. In hospital, these are usually plumbed in, but you can hire pools for use at home or you may be able to borrow one, if your local trust has the portable ones.

Ideally you should not enter the pool until you are in established labour. If you enter the pool too soon you may relax too well and stop the labour altogether! If the contractions are strong, however, and you need the pain relief offered by the water, you should get in. It is always helpful to check in advance what the policies are at your local unit, particularly if your partner would like to get in with you.

The midwife will monitor your labour as she would if you were not in the water, that is, she will check your temperature pulse and blood pressure at regular intervals, and listen to the baby's heart rate every 15–30 minutes. If there is not an underwater hand held doppler available, you may need to lift your bump out of the water for the midwife to hear the baby's heart beat. With an underwater doppler this will not be necessary.

The water should be kept at a fairly constant temperature, 36.5–37.5C, about normal body heat. If it is hotter than this, it is exhausting and may cause the baby's heart to beat too fast, if it is cooler, it will not give the benefits of the warmth. The water should be deep enough for you to be able to adopt whatever position you find comfortable.

It is better if you wear nothing in the pool, because a wet T-shirt, when exposed to the air, may leave you feeling cold. It is important that you have plenty of cold drinks available and you should also eat small amounts regularly so that you don't run out of energy.

Points to bear in mind:

- Some hospitals rule against using a birth pool if your pregnancy or labour is abnormal, e.g. pre-eclampsia, multiple pregnancy, or if your baby needs electronic heart monitoring. This doesn't say much for choice, so if you are planning to use a pool, discuss in advance about what may happen if you have problems in labour and, if possible, get the decisions in writing.

- As a rule, you will have more privacy if you are using a birth pool, as the pool rooms (or bathrooms) tend to be more isolated than ordinary rooms in labour wards. You should always have someone with you, however.

- You may have difficulty finding a midwife and/or hospital in your area who has waterbirth experience. If the local Director of Midwifery Services is unable to help, you may have to consider alternatives (go to a different hospital or GP unit, have a home birth, book an independent midwife) before you settle down to enjoy the rest of your pregnancy. Contact the local Community Health Council for advice on this issue.

- You are much more likely to be able to do your own thing, with a supportive midwife in a low-tech environment, for example at home, or in a small unit.

- You may have to pay to hire a pool – about £200 for four weeks hire.

- The water temperature has to be maintained. With a portable pool, this may mean your partner trotting back and forth with buckets to keep the temperature right!

- Many midwives would advise that you get into the pool when you are in established labour, that is to say, when your cervix is 4–5 cm dilated. Sometimes however, if labour is taking a long time to establish, you may find it helpful to rest and relax in the water.

- You can use some other forms of pain relief with water, such as traditional acupuncture, reflexology, massage, or entonox for example, but not TENS (obviously), pethidine (you may fall asleep and slip under the water) or an epidural (you need drips and monitors).

Other forms of pain relief

- **Acupuncture:** Acupuncture is an ancient Chinese healing technique. Very thin, fine needles are inserted into particular places on the body to produce a desired effect. As well as pain relief, acupuncture has also been used to turn breech babies and to induce labour. Responses vary from woman to woman, but most people find that, at minimum, it takes the edge off the contractions. The needles don't hurt, and there are no indications of adverse side effects.

- **Reflexology:** This is the art of applying pressure to particular areas of the feet or hands to produce healing, or, in the case of pregnancy and labour, the same conditions as acupuncture. There have been no reported adverse side effects, but it is more likely to be helpful if you have built up a rapport with the therapist.

- **Homoeopathy:** Homoeopathy works by treating 'like with like'. This means that minute doses of a substance are given which, if given at full strength, would cause the symptoms from which the patient is suffering. It's not quite that simple, though. The homoeopath needs to make an assessment of the sort of person you are, and how you are emotionally affected by your symptoms. If you are interested in having a homoeopath with you while you are in labour, she will bring her entire kit, as the remedies you need will alter according to progress and circumstance. You can buy 'labour kits' from homoeopathic retailers, with instructions, or a homoeopath may be willing to provide you with some remedies for specific events.

- **Hypnotherapy:** Hypnosis is very deep relaxation and requires a trained practitioner to work with you in order to achieve this relaxed state. You can be taught to hypnotise yourself (autohypnosis) or you can have a practitioner accompany you in labour. The longer you have to practise the techniques, the more effective it will be in controlling pain. It is worth noting that the research shows that one of the effects of hypnosis is to shorten the first stage of labour.

- **Aromatherapy:** Aromatherapists use the essential oils of plants to heal and soothe their clients. These oils have curative properties and have been used for thousands of years. Sometimes they are massaged into the skin, sometimes their essence is released in oil burners, or drops are put into a bath, or sprinkled on cloth and inhaled. Aromatherapists claim good results for the relief of pain in labour, as well as treatment for the minor disorders of pregnancy.

Make sure that you use qualified therapists, preferably recommended by someone you trust, and contact them early in your pregnancy. If you want to have a therapist with you while you are in labour, you should find out whether this will be acceptable to your midwife, or, if you are planning to go into hospital, check that there are no restrictions about who you bring with you. If you do this early enough, if gives you time to negotiate or make alternative arrangements.

You can phone the professional therapy organisations and ask them for a list of qualified practitioners in your area, or you may find such a list in the *Yellow Pages*.

7

Things that might go wrong

In this section, I've used technical terms, with explanations, so that you will be able to follow what's going on if any of these should happen to you.

POSITIONS OF THE BABY

The position of the baby in the uterus is called 'the lie'. This can be longitudinal, (which is either cephalic or breech), transverse, or oblique.

Cephalic (head down)

The normal position for the baby in the uterus is head down (Figure 7.1). The optimal position is with his back towards your front, and with his chin on his chest (flexed), which enables him to drop deep into the pelvis (engagement). This is called the 'occipito-anterior' position, which simply means that the back of the baby's head (the occiput) is facing your front. In this position, he can make his way through the birth canal easily and effectively. The contractions will be effective, because the pressure of the baby's head is spread evenly over the inside of the cervix, helping it to dilate; the membranes will not be subjected to uneven pressure and are more likely to stay intact; and the second stage will be quicker.

It sometimes happens that the baby's back is towards your back

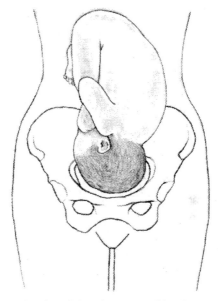

Figure 7.1 The optimal position for vaginal birth

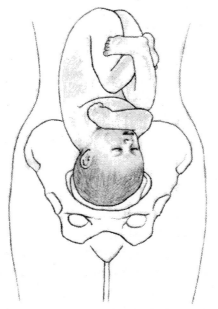

Figure 7.2 This baby is in the occipito-posterior position

(occipito-posterior) (Figure 7.2). In this position he is unable to flex his head and may not engage into your pelvis (called a 'high head'). The contractions will not be as effective, as the pressure of the baby's head will not be evenly distributed over the cervix. This can have a number of consequences, including:

- A long latent phase of labour

- Prolonged labour

- Early, spontaneous rupture of membranes, sometimes before labour starts

- Ineffective contractions

- Severe backache

- A pushing urge before the cervix is fully dilated, due to pressure of the back of the baby's head on the nerve plexus

- Higher incidence of epidural anaesthetic

- Higher incidence of forceps and ventouse deliveries

- Higher incidence of Caesarean section.

If your midwife tells you that the baby has his back to your back during the pregnancy, it may be possible to rectify it by exercises and appropriate movements. If this position is not diagnosed until you are in labour, then it is even more important that you are as upright and mobile as possible.

Breech (bottom down)

Lots of babies present as breech at some point during the pregnancy, but the vast majority will be head down by the time their mothers go into labour. About 3% will still be breech at term (Figure 7.3). If your baby is diagnosed as breech, and is still breech at 34 weeks, you may like to try pelvic tilts, which means lying down, raising your pelvis on a couple of pillows until it is higher than your head, pulling

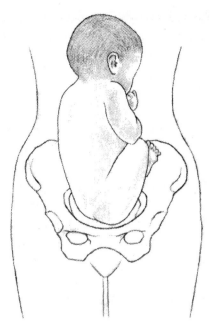

Figure 7.3 This baby is in the breech position. It is often recommended that a woman should be offered a Caesarean section for breech, but the evidence supporting normal (vaginal) breech delivery is quite favourable, depending on the way the baby is lying. See MIDIRS IC Leaflet *Breech presentation – options for care*

your thighs back towards your shoulders and breathing abdominally. You should do this for at least ten minutes at a time, so that you put in about a total of an hour a day.

It is now recommended by the Royal College of Obstetricians and Gynaecologists that a procedure called External Cephalic Version (ECV) should be attempted. You may be offered this, or you can ask for it. It is done by an obstetrician who manipulates your abdomen and gently pushes the baby into the right position. It isn't worth doing before 36 weeks and there is evidence to suggest that the closer to labour it is done, the more successful it is likely to be. You should also bear in mind that the ECV may be unsuccessful, or that the baby may return to his original position. If this happens, then your choice is still whether to have a vaginal delivery or a Caesarean.

You could also consult an acupuncturist, for a treatment called 'moxybustion' which is reported to have a good success rate at turning breech babies. Once you suspect that the baby has turned, whatever method you are using, stop all treatments and do some squatting every day, to encourage the head to go down into the pelvis.

It will probably be an obstetrician who discusses your options for delivery with you, as there are very few midwives (mostly independent), or doctors, who have the practice skills to deliver a breech baby routinely, although all are taught the theory and could do it in an emergency. There is plenty of evidence to suggest that in experienced hands, breech birth is a safe option, but you may have to find those experienced hands for yourself.

Many obstetricians would recommend a Caesarean section if it is your first baby and it is breech. This is for the following reasons:

• Increased risk of trauma to the baby, including bleeding into the brain (intracranial haemorrhage), fractures and dislocations of joints

• The risk of oxygen deficiency, due to compression of the cord

• The risk of trauma to the baby's nerves and muscles, particularly those in the neck and shoulder area

• There is some evidence to suggest that boys may have their fertility adversely affected due to bruising and swelling of the genitals.

• Your ability to push a baby out has not been established

• Lack of experience with vaginal breech births

Having said all that, you should know that many women labour with their firstborn breech babies without any ill effects, having found an experienced practitioner. It has been suggested that some of the above factors are due to professional inexperience and unless practitioners are able to gain that experience, there may come a time when all first babies presenting by the breech will be born by elective section.

Caesarean births are not without their own risks and you may not want to have one if it can be avoided. Ask for a second opinion, but check with other people, such as local branches of the National Childbirth Trust, to find out which obstetricians in the area are likely to be sympathetic to your wishes before you make an appointment.

With second or subsequent babies, if the first was of normal weight and gestation, the risks are reduced. You will have proved that your pelvis is adequate in size and that a baby can pass through it. Subsequent labours are also quicker, which means that your breech baby will be under less stress.

Oblique or transverse lie (lying across the uterus)

If either of these conditions persist, then vaginal delivery is impossible (Figure 7.4). For the baby to deliver vaginally, either the head or the breech should be presenting. With a transverse lie, it is usually the shoulder which blocks the way, although an oblique lie may correct itself when labour starts.

If your baby should be in either of these positions, you will be strongly advised to deliver in hospital. One reason is that if your waters break, there is a greater risk of cord prolapse, which is the umbilical cord coming through the cervix (there is no solid head or bottom in the way to prevent it). The other is that ECV (see above) may be advised. If that is unsuccessful, Caesarean section may well be necessary, as the baby will not be able to be born vaginally. Sometimes, however, contractions will push the baby into the right position, so it may be worth waiting until labour begins, but don't count on it.

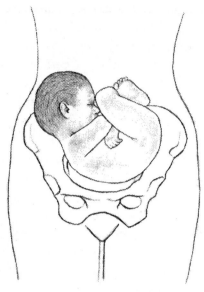

Figure 7.4 This baby is in the transverse position and will not be able to be born vaginally

Multiple pregnancy

When you are carrying twins or more, there are certain factors of which you should be aware before you make your choices. You may not suffer from any of these, but they are statistically more likely to happen:

- You may have a much greater degree of what are known as 'the minor disorders of pregnancy': sickness, tiredness, varicose veins, sleep disorders, backache, breathlessness.

- You are at greater risk of developing pregnancy induced hypertension.

- You are more likely to become anaemic.

- You are more at risk of antenatal bleeding and placenta praevia.

- You are more at risk of going into labour prematurely (before 37 weeks).

• The babies are more likely to be small and need special care.

Because of these risk factors you are likely to be advised to have your babies in a major hospital with a neonatal intensive care unit. Whether you will be advised to have a Caesarean section depends upon how many babies you are expecting, and how they are lying.

As far as twins are concerned, vaginal delivery appears to be a reasonable option. The research suggests there is nothing to gain in offering elective Caesareans to women expecting twins, but unfortunately, there appears to be very little research done into other aspects of delivering women with multiple pregnancies. If you are keen to give birth to your twins normally, and are meeting with resistance to this idea, or you want to have them at home, some independent midwives have a great deal of expertise in this field.

If you are expecting triplets, or more, the risks associated with vaginal delivery increase for the second and subsequent babies, so it is generally recommended, for their sake, that you have a section. The babies are likely to be small and may not stand up well to the rigours of labour. There is also a greater risk of placental separation once the membranes have ruptured, due to the sudden decrease in the size of the placental site on the wall of the uterus.

Placenta praevia

The placenta (afterbirth) is normally sited in the upper part of the uterus, well out of the way of the baby's passage into the vagina. In about 0.5–1% of women, however, the placenta will be in the lower part of the uterus, and in severe cases will cover the cervix on the inside. This means that if the woman were to go into labour, the placenta would come first, leaving the baby without an oxygen supply.

The degrees of severity are graded as follows:

1 Mostly in the upper part of the uterus, but with the edge coming into the lower part

2 Coming as far as, but not covering, the cervical canal (the 'os')

3 Partly covering the os

4 Completely covering the os.

Nobody knows why this should happen, but the following women are more at risk than others:

• Women who have given birth to more than four babies

• Multiple pregnancy (The placental area is much larger)

• Previous Caesarean section

• Smokers.

Having said that, it is still very uncommon even in these groups. Quite often women are told, after their 20 week scan, that the placenta is 'low' and that they will need a re-scan at 34 weeks. Most of these low placentae will be well out of the way by 34 weeks and no action will be needed.

The main danger associated with placenta praevia is bleeding. As the uterus grows, the placenta may begin to separate, which can give rise to quite heavy blood loss. The loss is painless and will start without any prior warning. Almost all serious cases of placenta praevia will be detected on scan and the woman will be advised about her options. In severe instances, the woman will be advised to come into hospital, where she will need to stay until the baby is delivered. Exactly when this will be is impossible to say, as it is dependent upon the degree of bleeding the woman experiences. If she has a serious episode, then the baby will be delivered by Caesarean section at that point. If she does not have any bleeding, then it is recommended that she has a Caesarean section before 38 weeks, as to risk going into labour could be disastrous.

If the placenta is just 'low', then a decision about the mode of delivery can be postponed until later in the pregnancy, when it can be seen whether the baby is able to get his head into the pelvis or not.

Pregnancy-induced hypertension (PIH or pre-eclampsia)

This is a syndrome which may possibly be some sort of immune disorder. The symptoms are a sharp rise in blood pressure, protein in the urine and oedema (water retention in the body tissues). The symptoms can sometimes reflect another condition; some women have higher blood pressure than others, without ill-effects; you may get protein in your urine if you have a urinary tract infection, or it can be due to contamination from vaginal discharge, so it is important to be certain of the exact cause. The third symptom of PIH, oedema, is less easy to assess. Almost all women have some degree of oedema, particularly in their feet, which is a sign of a healthy pregnancy, but in PIH this is extended to include swelling of some internal tissues as well. If the condition is severe, the tissues surrounding the liver and brain swell, causing the woman to have fits if not treated urgently. You should contact your midwife if you are concerned, particularly if you have headaches and/or visual disturbances such as bright flashing lights.

Some women will respond to treatment and bed rest in hospital, but those severely affected will need to be delivered, as this is the only cure. In the worst cases, the baby will need to be delivered by Caesarean section, which might have to be done well before the due date. The risks to the mother and baby of continuing the pregnancy, have to be balanced against the risks of delivering the baby early.

It is important to know that although you may have had PIH in an earlier pregnancy, you will not necessarily develop it next time. You should also be aware that if your baby has a different father, your chances of developing PIH are the same as with a first pregnancy.

Induction of labour

It is important to remember that no interventions in your labour can be carried out without your express consent. It has been shown that in many cases, one procedure will lead to another and to another, which has been called the cascade of intervention. You should be aware of how these procedures inter-relate.

Induction of labour is likely to be advised under the following circumstances:

- At about 41–42 weeks of pregnancy. There is a big difference in outcome between 41 and 42 weeks, and you may decide to wait until you have completed 41 weeks before considering induction[1].

- If your baby is not growing well, or has a condition requiring specialist help once he is born, then induction may well be recommended any time after about 34 weeks. It may even be before that, if the placenta is not functioning well, and, if so, the baby may fare better out than in.

- If you develop pregnancy-induced hypertension (PIH), there will come a point where for your sake and the baby's, it may be better to induce labour.

- If your waters break and you do not go into labour, most obstetricians would offer induction after 24 hours, although there is evidence to suggest that 90% of women will deliver within 72 hours. This is very much up to you.[1]

- If your baby is moving from one position to another, or is in the wrong position (breech, or even transverse) you may be offered the opportunity to be induced while the baby's position is stabilised (ECV – see above).

- If there is a pressing social reason – sometimes women whose partners are in the forces ask to be induced before their partner is posted overseas.

- If you have a medical condition which is being made worse by the continuation of the pregnancy.

- If the baby has a condition which indicates that delivery is in his best interests, whatever the stage of the pregnancy. This can include certain blood disorders, in particular Rhesus incompatibility, which can occur (but very rarely these days) when a Rhesus negative woman is carrying a Rhesus positive baby.

As with all other interventions, you have a right to be fully informed, with particular regard to your individual circumstances. You should be able to discuss all the advantages and disadvantages before you make up your mind one way or the other. Don't agree to be induced until you have thoroughly explored all the options.

You should be aware that induction is not without its own risk factors. You have a greater chance of:

- Caesarean section

- instrumental delivery

- epidural anaesthetic

- infection

- episiotomy

- a longer hospital stay.

All these need to be considered before you make up your mind.

Measures which can be taken to bring on labour through artificial means include:

- rupture of the membranes (ARM)

- the use of prostaglandin intravaginally

- an intravenous infusion (IV, or a 'drip') of syntocinon (a synthetic version of the hormone oxytocin, which makes the uterus contract)

- a combination of the three.

1. Breaking the waters/artificial rupture of the membranes (ARM)

There has been a history of routine ARM being practised once established labour has been diagnosed, (most often defined when the cervix was 3 or more centimetres dilated). This was most often performed by the midwife, or on occasion, by an obstetrician. You should know that once the membranes have been ruptured, you are irrevocably committed to delivery, as the risk of infection ascending into the uterus, and consequently to the baby, increases, the longer the membranes are ruptured.

The reasons most often given for artificially rupturing the membranes are:

- to speed up or augment the labour, thereby shortening the length of time before the baby's birth

- to monitor the colour of the liquor

- to apply a fetal scalp electrode (FSE) to the baby's scalp to monitor his heart rate continuously using a cardiotocograph (CTG) machine.

There are several points you may wish to consider before consenting to an ARM being performed.

- An ARM may speed up your labour, shortening it by up to two hours if it is performed appropriately. However many women find there is an immediate, sharp increase in pain of contractions associated with ARM. This may necessitate the administration of pain relief, which you may have been able to do without, if you had built up to that point gradually.

- If you are in spontaneous labour and the baby's heart rate is listened to intermittently with either a Pinard stethoscope (ear trumpet) or Doppler ultrasound (a hand held monitor), and it is within the expected 'normal' limits, there is no evidence to support performing an ARM.

- If your labour is progressing, is not taking an unusually long time and your baby is not showing signs of becoming tired or 'distressed', it is unlikely that an ARM will help.

- If your labour is progressing slowly, there may be other more helpful things that could be done first, such as mobilising, changing position, having something to drink and a light, high energy food to eat. You may find it helpful to dim the lights and take time out to relax and recoup your energy. If the baby's heart rate is within the expected 'normal' limits, there is no reason to put an arbitrary time limit on your labour.

If there is evidence of your baby becoming tired or distressed, it may be prudent to have an ARM for assessment of the liquor. If you have been lying in bed, however, you may find that, by mobilising, your baby will be much happier and your labour may progress much more quickly.

In order to perform an ARM, your midwife will need to perform a vaginal examination. She will need to assess the dilatation of the cervix, the position of the baby's head in relation to your pelvis and how well the baby's head is applied to (i.e. how well it is resting against) the cervix. Once she has satisfied herself that all is favourable, and that the cervix is sufficiently dilated, she will then rupture the membranes using an instrument like a plastic crochet-hook, called an amnihook. The procedure is generally no more unpleasant than any vaginal examination can be for women, although if the cervix is only 3 centimetres dilated and the procedure is difficult for the midwife or obstetrician to perform, the examination can cause distress and pain for the woman. With current knowledge of the few, if any benefits, of performing an ARM early in labour and the probable negative effects to both the woman and her baby this may cause, there would be few instances when a midwife or obstetrician would perform ARM routinely.

2. Prostaglandin gel

The more effaced and dilated (ripe) the cervix is, the more likely it is that ARM will be successful on its own. If, however, the cervix is not ripe, then prostaglandin gel will be recommended. Prostaglandin ripens the cervix and for many women will serve as a 'kick-start' into labour.

The gel (or sometimes a pessary) is introduced into the vagina as high as possible, around the cervix. The woman is then strapped to a monitor for an hour or so to assess the effect of the attempted induction on the baby. If all is well, she will then be encouraged to walk around and wait for contractions to start.

The contractions produced by the prostaglandin may be short, but quite sharp at the beginning, so use breathing, relaxation and positions to deal with them. In many instances, these contractions will gradually lengthen into proper labour contractions and all will proceed normally without further interventions being required. Sometimes, two or more doses may be needed before a result, but all in all, it is a less intrusive method of induction than a drip.

3. Intravenous syntocinon

Syntocinon is given directly into a vein in very small doses, which are very carefully calculated. Too much can put the uterus into spasm; too little will be ineffective. It is always done in hospital and you will need to be constantly monitored to assess the effect the process is having on the baby and on the uterus. Some babies simply do not respond well to induction, and Caesarean section may be necessary.

Some hospitals connect the IV containing the syntocinon to a bag of intravenous fluid, usually a salt and sugar solution. This enables the IV to run constantly (the main bag is renewed when it empties) and prevents the vein from closing up, as the volume of syntocinon is so low. Other hospitals use a continuous pump into the vein which runs very slowly at a pre-set amount, using an even lower dose. This has the advantage of keeping down the volume of fluid put into the bloodstream.

The dose starts at a low rate and is gradually increased until the contractions are coming every two minutes. There is no gradual build-up to the contractions, so there is no chance to acclimatise yourself to them. Many women being induced choose to have an epidural for this reason. If you decide to do this, then the epidural will be sited before the syntocinon is started. Once the baby is born, the drip is usually maintained for a while, as there is always the risk that having artificially stimulated the uterus, it may relax if the stimulation is stopped too quickly, which would lead to heavy bleeding.

Augmentation of labour

This is similar to induction, but it is the procedure which is used if labour has already begun. Reasons why it may be recommended include:

- Ineffectual/irregular contractions
- Prolonged labour
- Slow progress once labour is established.

Sometimes the body finds it difficult to actually establish contractions that will dilate the cervix. Mobilisation and taking food and drink may sometimes be enough to get things going, but not always.

All the procedures, drugs, etc., are the same as for induction, and, as before, you have to consent to the procedure, so make sure that you have all the information you need. You should also take time to ask questions and discuss it with your birth partner before you decide.

Non-invasive methods of induction

This covers a number of different options, from herbalism and homoeopathy to acupuncture and reflexology. Whichever therapy (or therapies) you decide to try, ring around first. Always choose a reputable practitioner with appropriate qualifications who is a member of a national body. These national organisations will be only too pleased to tell you what qualifications are relevant to their speciality. You might also ask friends and acquaintances whether they could recommend someone who is experienced in this area – they do exist.

Everybody knows that having sex can also bring on labour (semen contains prostaglandin), but what is less well known is that female orgasm is pretty good at getting contractions going, so masturbation can sometimes help if your induction date is looming. Nipple stimulation can also get contractions started, or get them going again if they have gone off a bit, and has the advantage that you can do it in a hospital room! Do be aware, however, that none of these will get labour going unless you, your body and the baby are ready.

Fetal distress

In labour your uterus acts like a piston and with each contraction your baby will be moved more into your pelvis and eventually to birth. The power of your uterus is remarkable, and, unlike any other muscle in your body, after each contraction it will not relax back to the size it was before, but will slowly decrease the size of the space in which your baby has lived since shortly after conception. This will, of course, give him little option other than to go further down into your pelvis. In most pregnancies, the placenta will find itself a secure place in the upper part of your uterus, known as the fundus. As the baby is pushed through your pelvis with each contraction, your placenta remains at the fundus and is also subjected to the pressure of each contraction.

With each contraction, there will be a decrease in oxygen and nutrient-rich blood from your circulation reaching the fine membranes of the placenta, where it is transported across to your baby's circulatory system. Under normal labour conditions your baby will not be unduly affected by this and will be able to cope perfectly well.

Your midwife should keep you fully informed of any concerns she may have with regard to your progress in labour, or your baby's ability to cope with the labour, which may be indicated by changes in his heart rate, which is evidence of fetal distress. You should try to be mobile and in an upright position, as this will make it easier for your baby to get enough oxygen and it will help with the progress of your labour. If you are already upright you should try and change your position, especially if you have been in one position for some time. You may find that you have an urge to adopt a particular position – listen to what your body is telling you and try to go with it.

In the situation where a baby is, for some reason, compromised, the heart rate baseline will usually drop (bradycardia). For a baby that is stressed by labour, or compromised, a normal central nervous system response is for him to open his bowels and pass meconium. Other signs that a baby is possibly compromised include a decrease in the heart rate after contractions (late decelerations), a flattening out of the heart rate (loss of beat-to-beat variability) and sometimes a high baseline heart rate (tachycardia). Loss of contact with the monitor's electrode is not a sign of fetal distress!

Electronic fetal heart monitoring

There is no evidence to support Continuous Electronic Fetal Monitoring (CEFM or EFM) with a cardiotocographic (CTG) trace in normal, spontaneous labour. The research evidence clearly shows that a midwife listening regularly to the fetal heart (every twenty minutes or so) is reliable, less invasive and less subject to false alarms.

A normal fetal heart rate usually increases when the baby kicks, or at the beginning of a contraction, and drops back to the 'normal' baseline at the end of the contraction or when he stops moving. A heart-beat that does this is called 'reactive'. All babies have regular quiet periods, or sleep times, when the heart rate settles to a slower, less reactive pattern.

If your labour is induced, or you have an epidural and/or your baby shows signs of becoming distressed, a continuous CTG may be needed. The only indication to apply a Fetal Scalp Electrode (FSE) is if the abdominal transducer is not picking up a good, readable trace. This may be because of the baby's position, or sometimes, if the woman is very overweight, it can be difficult to get a clear recording.

The scalp electrode is passed into the vagina and attached to the skin of the baby's scalp at one end. The other end is connected to the monitor and is fastened to the woman's thigh with a length of elastic, like a garter. Some FSEs are sharp needles which clip into the top layer of the baby's scalp, and some (newer) are little suction cups. There is no doubt that the suction is gentler and less invasive – you may like to find out which hospitals in your area use which types of FSE.

A fetal scalp electrode and repeated vaginal examinations, no matter how careful your midwife or obstetrician, may put you and your baby at a greater risk of infection.

Meconium stained liquor

Around 12 weeks following conception, your baby will begin to suck and swallow the liquor around him (amniotic fluid). Although his digestive tract is largely unused, he will already have almost all of his gastric juices, which will be fully utilised after birth, when he receives his nutrition from milk. From the moment that he begins to swallow, however, he will consume any debris that is in the liquor, including skin cells that have been shed from his body and digestive tract. Your baby's gastric juices will act on these and the end result will be meco-nium – the baby's first bowel movement – which in most babies remains in their digestive system until after birth. Meconium is described as a thick, tenacious, greenish-black substance (somewhere between tar and silage) which is usually passed in large amounts in the first 48 hours following his birth and is something with which you will become an expert at dealing!

Meconium may be passed without any evidence of cause in some babies before their birth. It may even be passed prior to labour commencing. A baby that passes meconium in the presence of good amounts of liquor and is not showing any adverse effects from the labour or birth process is unlikely to be in danger. This is classically seen as a thin brown to green discolouring of the liquor and is thought to be due, very simply, to the bowel being full!

Your midwife will check any meconium in the liquor, and its consistency, in order to classify the amount, the thickness and type. This is often done in graduation from 1–4. For example, grade 1 meconium is thinly mixed in good quantities of liquor and grade 4 is thick fresh meconium with little evidence of liquor. (In all pregnancies it is normal for the liquor volume to begin to lessen in quantity from around 37 weeks.) The greater the gradation of, or the thicker, the meconium the greater the risk to your baby and the more probable it is that he will show signs of being tired and fatigued by the birth process.

Meconium passed during the process of labour and birth may be caused by the baby being unable to receive enough oxygen. Most babies begin labour with good reserves and an ability to cope with the demands and stresses placed on them. When labour is at term, spontaneous in onset, and there are no other irregularities, there is no evidence to suggest that your baby will have difficulty in receiving enough oxygen.

If the passing of meconium results in, or is associated with, your baby's heart rate reducing, particularly at the end of or after the contraction has passed (late decelerations), this is an indication that your baby may need assistance to birth soon. The danger for the baby is that he will try to gasp for breath and thereby take meconium into his lungs.

Meconium aspiration (meconium breathed into the lungs) can cause serious medical complications for your baby. It is highly probable that in the presence of apnoea (lack of oxygen), evidenced by classic changes in his heart rate and the passage of meconium, a paediatrician will be present and the birth will be accelerated. The paediatrician will as soon as possible want to gently examine the baby's throat, larynx and lungs, using an instrument called a laryngoscope. This examination can take place before the cord is cut and you may want to consider this.

It may be reassuring for you to remember that there is evidence that a well baby, who begins the birth process with a spontaneous labour, will only attempt to breathe or gasp in the uterus if severely compromised through a lack of oxygen.

If your baby requires any active help and assistance at birth, leaving the cord intact may well provide him with a few minutes of oxygenated and nutrient rich blood from the placenta. While your placenta is still able to supply oxygen and nutrients, and collect the baby's waste, he will benefit. The combination of placenta, midwife and paediatrician assistance can give your baby a better start.

Obviously the type of birth and the degree of emergency will affect whether or not the cord can be left to pulsate and provide your baby with extra help and time to adjust. (See later section on cutting the cord.) If there is any indication that the presence of a paediatrician will be required in advance, it may be a good idea to discuss with him leaving the cord intact for the first few minutes and any examination being done at your side.

Fetal blood sampling

If your baby does exhibit signs of distress, then you may be advised to have this procedure, which is normally carried out by an obstetrician. The more distressed a baby is, the more acid his blood, so a droplet of blood is taken to measure the acid level. If all seems well, you can carry on as normal. If it is dubious, then you will be advised to have your labour more closely monitored, with another blood sampling done within a specified period of time. If the blood shows that the baby is acidotic, then you will be advised to have a Caesarean section, or, if the baby is nearly born, then instrumental delivery will be recommended.

In order to obtain the blood sample from the baby, you will have to have your membranes ruptured. Then, an accessible area of the baby's head will be given a little burst of a cold spray which helps to bring blood to the vessels in that area. A very small incision is made and the droplet that forms is collected in a thin tube called a capillary tube. The blood acid levels are measured immediately and the decision made is based upon the findings there and then.

EPISIOTOMY

An episiotomy is a cut, made at the end of the vaginal entrance into the perineum, to widen the outlet. Some women will be advised to have an episiotomy to assist and expedite the birth of the baby, if there are indications of severe distress. However episiotomies may be performed under other circumstances, for example when forceps are used or if the baby is premature, to protect his delicate head.

It used to be the case that most first-time mothers were given an episiotomy routinely, in the mistaken belief that it would make things easier and save strain on the pelvic floor, but this is no longer so. It is still first-timers who are most likely to have an episiotomy, but midwives are now aware that this surgical intervention should never be done routinely and are also aware of the importance of discussing the reason why it may be necessary.

These days, midwives are more aware of the importance of a slow emergence of the baby's head and are likely to encourage you to 'breathe the head out' rather than pushing as hard as you can. Breathing through the contractions means a lot of concentration and support, so antenatal classes can be very helpful in practising these techniques. Different positions can also help to reduce the strain on the perineum – all fours and kneeling in particular.

Avoiding an episiotomy is an issue which is of major importance to many women. The sort of skin you have tells how well your perineum will stretch to accommodate the delivery of the baby. If you have lots of stretch marks and you are only expecting one, normal sized baby, then you may find that your skin is not very elastic. You can try perineal massage: using a natural oil (sweet almond is good, but be very careful if you have an allergy to nuts) pour a little into the palm of your hand to warm it. Then, dip your thumb into the oil. Using a side to side movement, press gently on the perineum in the direction of the anus and do this for a minute or so, until it feels stretched. Then, dip your thumb and forefinger in the remains of the oil, and using a circular, pinching movement, stretch the perineum outwards, again until you get the feeling of being stretched. Do this every day from about 30 weeks onwards – if nothing else, it will acclimatise you to the stretching sensations you feel when the baby is being born.

1 *Guide to Effective Care in Pregnancy and Childbirth*

8

Giving birth

Your labour may not go the way you planned. You may have booked a homebirth and had to transfer to hospital, or your midwife may have been looking after someone else and you have had to have a midwife you don't know. The important thing, however, is to have aspirations rather than expectations. That way, you avoid the let-down feeling which some women have when the event does not follow the birth plan.

Expect to be supported in your choices, and enlist the active support of your birth partner. The need for assertiveness should only arise if you feel you are being obstructed by those caring for you. It is, after all, you who is having this baby and you have every right to deliver your baby in the way which is best for you both.

Unless you know the midwife caring for you, a relationship, based on mutual respect, must be established in a relatively short space of time; the midwife's respect for your informed decisions, and yours for her professionalism.

It can be appallingly difficult to challenge somebody if you have not been given all the information, so if you don't understand what's going on, ask questions (or get your partner to do so) until you do understand. Then you can make your decision.

Finally, if you believe that you and the midwife or doctor will not be able to reach agreement on an issue which is important to you, then you can ask to have someone else to look after you. Try to keep it civil, but be firm. You won't get another go at having this baby, so it should be as right as you can make it.

The second stage

The second stage of labour is measured in terms of 'progress', that is, the gradual descent of the baby's head. As long as progress is being made, then the time it takes is, to a large extent, irrelevant. Some women will push their first babies out in half an hour, others may take two or three hours, but take heart. Subsequent babies will usually only take a few minutes. The research shows that setting arbitrary time limits, such as an hour for a first baby and half an hour for a second, are neither helpful, nor realistic. If you are having your baby in a place where these limits are set, even if everything else is normal, then you are entitled to say that you don't want any intervention and to have your decision respected. If a policy can't be backed by appropriate research, then it constitutes a prejudice, not a reasoned judgement. Try to find out in advance whether such policies exist where you plan to have your baby, or discuss your preferences with your midwife.

Once the cervix has fully dilated, there may be an interval while the contractions stop. As long as the baby is showing no signs of distress, then just rest and be thankful. The midwife may suggest an internal examination to confirm that your cervix is fully dilated. If you have no urge to push, and everything else is fine, then there is nothing to be gained by trying; just wait until the contractions start again and you will probably find the urge is there.

Pushing

Sometimes people will try to encourage you to push as soon as your cervix is fully dilated. Do be clear and say that you don't feel like pushing yet. You'll run the risk of exhausting yourself, so let your

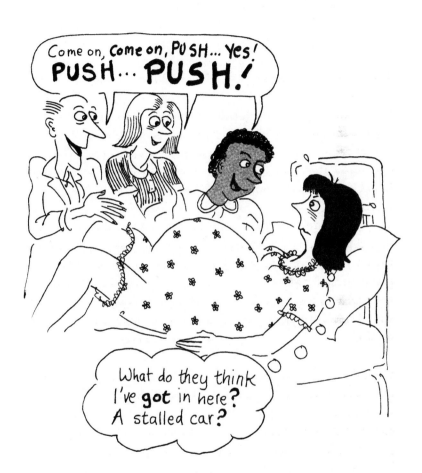

body do the hard work, while you wait until it's time to join in. The research evidence shows that pushing when your body feels the urge is more efficient in birthing the baby, and does not compromise his oxygen intake. It is of no benefit to be told to hold your breath, grit your teeth and bear down. Left to themselves, women will let the breath out with an open throat while pushing, which is more effective. You will make funny noises, grunts and gasps. Some women find it helps to shout or scream – go with it. Whatever works!

If you have had pethidine, then concentration can be a problem. It can also interfere with the way in which your body and mind communicate – you may not interpret the signals correctly because you feel very sleepy. Under these circumstances, you may find clear directions from someone very helpful, but otherwise be guided by your physical sensations.

Many women are encouraged to lie, propped up, either with their feet in the air, or flat on the bed. This is not an optimal position. Let gravity do its job – an upright position, as the diagrams show, will help you. Visualise where the baby is, where he's going to emerge and direct the force of your push to that point. Ask your birth partner to help you move to a useful position, as you will have discussed at classes.

Some women feel frightened as the baby moves down, as if they are going to tear themselves. The baby can feel enormous at this point, but the situation is a bit like when you have a hole in your tooth – it feels massive, but when you look in the mirror, there's nothing to be seen! Be comforted in knowing that you are perfectly designed to get a baby through your vagina. Your midwife is there to help you and the baby cope with what is happening. If you are distressed by the burning sensations as the baby's head comes to the vaginal entrance, hot compresses on the perineum can be very helpful at this point.

If you are in a birthing pool, then moving is much easier and you are less likely to be pressured into a particular delivery position. Some women find the resistance of the water helps with pushing, but others find it easier out of the water, so be prepared to move out if it doesn't feel right. You will also be advised to leave the pool if there is evidence of fetal distress, such as meconium stained liquor, or if the heartbeat is abnormal.

It used to be thought beneficial for the midwife to press firmly on the baby's head as it emerged, to control it, so it was easiest for her if her clients were lying down. We now know from the research that this pressure makes no difference, but that delivering the head slowly does. Instead of pressing the baby's head, the midwife is more likely to watch your perineum carefully, advise you on your breathing and keep a hand lightly on the top of his head as it emerges. As a result, many more midwives are encouraging women to adopt what used to be called alternative positions – that is, anything which isn't lying on your back in bed!

If this is not your first baby, then you may find that the urge to push is stronger than with your first. If the urge is very strong, then you may find it helpful to try to 'breathe through' the contractions, in order to control the rate at which the baby arrives. Do this by blowing your breath out and concentrating on that, rather than letting yourself hold your breath to bear down. If things are progressing very quickly, then it may be useful to adopt the 'knee-chest position' which will give you a measure of control over it.

Long pushes are not more effective than short ones – what is important is to capitalise upon each push's progress. It's a bit like rolling a boulder up a slope; you stop, take a breath, push again, hold the boulder there, take a breath, push again.

You will find that some contractions are 'pushier' than others, but you will get 3–5 pushes with a strong contraction, each lasting about 6 seconds. The baby will come down a little with each push then slip back, but not completely, at the end of the contraction, gradually opening up the vagina, and with his head gently moulding to ease his passage. This moulding usually disappears within 24 hours, so there's no need to be concerned if his head is an odd shape.

Positions for normal labour

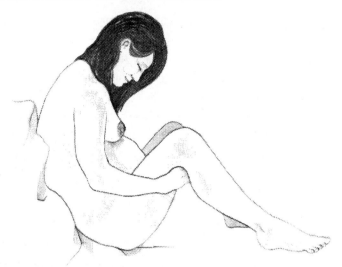

Figure 8.1 A position often adopted in hospital. Disadvantages are that the direction of push is 'uphill' and the pelvis is unable to expand because you're sitting on it!

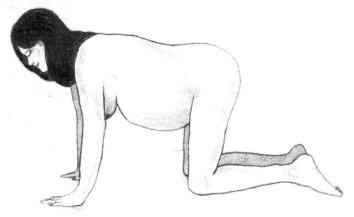

Figure 8.2 In an upright position, on all-fours (as here), kneeling, or standing supported, the pelvis can open and gravity helps

Waterbirths

If there are no problems during labour, you may decide to stay in the water for the birth. You will find changing position much easier in the water and pushing is a more controlled process, due to the counter-pressure of the water.

Once the baby is born, you can reach down and bring him to the surface straight away. The baby's body should be kept in the warm water to prevent him getting cold, but his head should never go back under the water once he has been brought to the surface.

The umbilical cord is not cut until you leave the pool for the delivery of the placenta. Many women choose to stay in the pool for a while with the baby, perhaps even to give him a feed while waiting for signs that the third stage is about to begin (see below).

Research into the safety of waterbirths has been conducted by the National Perinatal Epidemiology Unit in Oxford. The survey was commissioned by the Department of Health in response to a recommendation by the Commons Select Committee that all hospitals should provide pools where practicable. The research suggests that labour and birth in water are safe options for women with normal pregnancies and labours.

You should however, keep your mind open to change. If, for some reason, (possibly slow progress, or fetal distress) you are asked to leave the water, you run the risk of being very disappointed that you did not achieve your waterbirth. You should also consider that if the baby does become distressed, or is too cold, he stands a greater chance of gasping under the water. It may also take longer to get help if it's needed, as you will have to get out of the water and other problems, such as the fetal heart rate, may take longer to be diagnosed.

Positions with an epidural

If you have an epidural, you are limited in the birth positions you can
choose. This is partly because, if you have a full epidural, you won't
be able to use your legs, partly because you will be attached to a fetal
heart monitor and partly because any sort of epidural affects the
joints and ligaments of the pelvis and spine. These joints become
more relaxed than they are normally, so it is easy to damage them if
they are over-extended. You should always be lifted properly by two
people and never let yourself be dragged into position.

The following positions are suitable for a full epidural. If you have a
mobile epidural be very careful of your pelvis and lower back while
sensation is absent. Good positions for delivery are lying on your left
side and possibly a squatting position on the bed with someone to
support on either side.

Instrumental (operative) deliveries

With the best will in the world, sometimes it becomes necessary to
help the baby out:

- if he is distressed

- if you are exhausted

- if he has turned awkwardly in the pelvis

- if he stays in the occipito-posterior position and cannot turn
  himself.

In this case, you will need forceps or ventouse to deliver him. The
procedure should be performed by a doctor who has been trained to
do this, or who is being supervised and is at least a registrar. In order
for an instrumental delivery to take place, your cervix must be fully
dilated and you should have effective pain relief in place. In most circumstances, if there is time, you would be advised to have an
epidural, but if the baby is nearly there, some doctors recommend a

'pudendal block', which is local anaesthetic into the pudendal nerve at the top of the vagina.

The forceps are slid, one blade at a time, into the vagina and grasp the baby's head on either side. With the handles locked together, the doctor pulls as you push. A ventouse is attached to the baby's head by vacuum and, again, the operator pulls as you push.

If you need to have an instrumental delivery, it could be in your, and your baby's, best interests to ask if a ventouse could be used rather than forceps. The research suggests that in almost all cases a ventouse is preferable to forceps, as it is less likely to cause injury to mother and baby, needs less analgesia and can be used wherever forceps are used. You should be aware, though, that the efficiency of the ventouse is dependent upon the skill of the operator. Whilst its use is widespread on the continent, it is not so well known here, although increasingly, doctors are aware of the advantages and are becoming proficient.

Caesarean sections (LSCS)

Caesarean Sections constitute major abdominal surgery and the reasons for doing such surgery are divided into two groups – elective, that is, decided upon in advance, and emergency.

Elective sections

Reasons given for recommending elective sections:

- placenta praevia (see Chapter 7)
- a baby lying across the uterus who refuses to move (transverse lie)
- severe pre-eclampsia in the mother
- a baby who is too little or too ill to risk labour
- a pre-existing maternal illness, such as heart disease, which would make labour ill-advised

- active genital herpes (if the lesions are not active, vaginal birth is a safe option)

- multiple pregnancies, but not necessarily twins.

The following reasons can be negotiated, as the research indicates that sections are not always necessary in these circumstances:

1 the baby is thought to be too big to pass through the pelvis

2 a breech baby

3 twins (it depends upon the way the babies are lying).

In reason 1, the pelvic joints can be quite stretchy in labour. It is not yet possible to be completely accurate about a baby's size, even with a scan, so the only way to see if this baby will be born vaginally is to find out through progress in labour. For a discussion of reasons 2 and 3, see Chapter 7.

If you disagree with a proposed course of action, you are always entitled to ask for a second opinion. It may be, for example, that you are happy with the decision to have a section, but you would prefer to go into labour before having the operation, and the consultant does not agree. If you are unable to negotiate a settlement which both of you regard as satisfactory, then before you ask for a second opinion, ask around local contacts as to which obstetrician at which hospital is likely to be flexible in his or her views.

Emergency sections

Reasons for emergency sections are:

- fetal distress

- sudden, severe bleeding with placental separation

- cord prolapse (a rare situation, where a loop of cord comes through the cervix ahead of the baby. The resulting compression of the cord can be fatal to him)

- a cervix which doesn't dilate, in spite of interventions to make contractions effective and regular

- a baby which doesn't come down through the pelvis when the cervix is fully dilated, in spite of pushing, or even with forceps

- a sudden deterioration in the mother's wellbeing

- sudden, severe pre-eclampsia.

If a section is needed, you should be fully informed about what is going on. It is still your decision whether to undergo surgery and you have to sign a form, specifically giving your consent to the procedure. If you don't understand, ask questions until you do; take a support person with you if an elective section is being recommended and don't decide there and then. Go home, discuss it with your partner, your midwife, your GP, and anyone else you think may have a useful opinion. Then decide. If you are in labour, of course, the time scale is a bit different, but even so you should be fully informed about what is happening, why a section is considered necessary and what the consequences are likely to be if you wait, or decide not to have the operation. There have been instances in the past when women have been forcibly sectioned, but the courts now take a very dim view of this and it is illegal to perform this action on a person who is deemed capable of making her own decisions.

With elective sections, you can generally decide whether you would prefer to have a general anaesthetic or an epidural. Most anaesthetists would recommend an epidural, as recovery is quicker, you can feed the baby as soon as you like and you feel that you have been present at your baby's birth. You may feel however, that it would not suit you to be awake whilst you are being operated on, and would prefer to wake up when it's all over.

Vaginal birth after caesarean section (VBAC)

It is commonly believed that having had a Caesarean section constitutes a 'risk' for future labours, which means giving birth under the care of a consultant in a hospital. A 'trial of labour' is set up to ensure a quick and easy transfer to the operating theatre if an emergency happens. This is due to the mistaken belief that the previous scar on the uterus has a high chance of rupture, with catastrophic consequences. Some women, as well as some doctors and midwives, feel that this may not necessarily be the best option and the evidence supports that belief.

The key issues are what sort of incision was used and why the previous section was done. The research shows that vaginal birth after a Caesarean section (VBAC) is a safe option for women with a lower segment (horizontal) scar. You should also know that the risk of damage to the uterus after one section of this kind is only fractionally higher than for a woman who has never had a section. The risk does increase after two sections, but even so, it is small enough for the *Guide to Effective Care in Pregnancy and Childbirth* to say,

'The available evidence does not suggest that a woman who has had more than one previous lower segment Caesarean section should be treated any differently from the woman who has had only one.'

The other type of incision is a 'classical' incision, which runs vertically down the abdomen. With this type of scar, the research indicates that the risks of rupture are much higher – four times higher, in fact. This incision is very rarely done these days, but may be done, if, for example, a section is performed early in pregnancy, or if fibroids need to be removed. Under these circumstances, an elective section in subsequent pregnancies would seem to be, at least, a course of action which should be seriously considered.

As far as reasons for the previous section are concerned, if you had a section for fetal distress, your chances of a normal delivery next time appear to be about 68%. If your previous section was because the baby was breech or transverse, the VBAC rate is about 73%. If you had a section for 'failure to progress' or slow progress, then the chances vary depending, apparently, upon the degree of cervical dilatation you reached before the section was performed. If it was 5cm or less, then your chances are calculated at 67%. If it was 6–9cm the success rate is 73%, but if your cervix was fully dilated, then the rate drops to 13%. These are all factors that you need to put into the equation when you are deciding whether to go into labour or whether to have an elective section. Women who go into labour naturally stand a far better chance of a vaginal delivery than those who have their labour induced. Once in labour, it has been shown that women in hospitals who are given a longer time to labour, and who are encouraged to be upright and active, are more likely to give birth vaginally.

There is no research evidence to support the practice of putting in intravenous needles 'just in case', nor for continuous electronic fetal monitoring without a specific clinical reason. Given the findings, you may well decide that you prefer not to have such interventions. The *Guide to Effective Care in Pregnancy and Childbirth*, says, 'The care of a woman in labour after a previous lower segment Caesarean section should be little different from that of any woman in labour.'

Childbirth is a social and personal experience as well as being considered a medical event. Some people have in the past suggested that a woman who wants a normal birth after a section is putting her own needs before her baby's. This is untrue and unfair. A woman's natural instinct is to protect her baby at all costs; its safety and wellbeing are her prime concern. She must also consider her own needs, however, and be aware that a normal delivery is much more likely if she knows what will help her, and if she is confident in her own ability.

The third stage

The third stage of labour is the delivery of the placenta and membranes. In the old days, it used to be a time of great anxiety for the midwife, as this was the time when a woman could bleed very seriously. This was primarily due to the fact that without contraception, women were producing babies every eighteen months or so. As a result of this, and poor diet, they were exhausted, anaemic and prone to infections, all of which predisposed them to haemorrhage.

We now have contraception, good public health (due to the innovation of the closed sewage system) and the highest level of nutrition in this country ever. The historical dread of postnatal haemorrhage is still present within the professions, however, and this fear has lead to a system of care in the third stage which, these days, is not always appropriate.

As the uterus contracts after the birth, the internal dimensions of the uterus are reduced, and the placenta shears off the wall. There is a small amount of blood loss, which indicates that the placenta is separating. If left to itself, particularly with the woman in an upright position, there will be a further contraction, together with an urge to push, and the placenta is delivered. The uterus is then able to contract tightly, preventing further blood loss, apart from the normal loss which goes on for several days after the birth. The third stage can also be helped along by putting the baby to the breast, or stimulating the nipples; these actions release the hormone oxytocin, causing the uterus to contract.

The cord can be cut at any point, but it is usual to wait until it has stopped pulsating, as this indicates that the placenta has ceased to function. Your partner may like to cut the cord.

This method of dealing with the third stage is called, physiological, or natural, third stage. In women who have had normal labours and births, without augmentation or instrumental delivery, it is a safe option. The research evidence is clear that where experienced practitioners, using accepted criteria, manage the third stage physiologically, the outcomes are safe.

Most women in hospitals are given an injection to cause the uterus to contract down hard. This acts to produce a sustained contraction, starting within 5 minutes of administration and lasting for about an hour and a half. The injection is usually given as the baby's shoulders are born, and it is called syntometrine. It comprises two separate elements: syntocinon, which is the drug used to induce and augment labour, and ergometrine, which is a synthetic form of ergot. (Interestingly, ergot, which is derived from a mould which grows on rye, used to be used by witches to induce hallucinations of flying! It has been given by midwives to women for thousands of years). Once you have had the injection, the cord must be clamped and cut to prevent the baby getting a sudden rush of blood when the uterus contracts.

Ergometrine in particular has side effects which you may like to take into account when making your decisions about how you would like to manage your third stage:

• nausea and vomiting

• a rise in blood pressure

• pains in the muscles of the inner thighs.

It doesn't only contract the muscles of the uterus, it contracts all smooth muscle, including the stomach, the small muscles round blood vessels and the thigh muscles, hence these side effects. If you have raised blood pressure, you will be given syntocinon on its own, rather than risk the possibility of increasing the blood pressure with ergometrine.

Once the uterus has contracted, the midwife will put her hand on your abdomen, over the uterus, and press firmly in an upwards and backwards direction. She will then grasp the cord and pull the placenta out. The advantage of an actively managed third stage is that it only takes about 5 minutes, as compared to a physiological one, which can take up to an hour. There are no drug-induced side effects with a physiological third stage, however, and many women feel that this is a good enough reason for avoiding active management of the third stage where possible.

9

Birth reports

On the last pages, you will find some birth stories. Some of them went as planned, and some didn't, but these women feel good about their experiences and want to share them. After you have had your baby, you need to share your experiences too. All too often we hear of women going about their lives in silence, feeling that they should just get on with it – and how come we never hear the good stories? Talk about your experiences; share them and encourage others to do the same. In this way, networks of support and expertise are built up that benefit us all and will empower and encourage our daughters in their turn.

If this book has only given you the basis for a birth plan, then that's good enough. I hope, though, that it has given you much more than that. I would like to think that it has given you the information you need to ensure that all your decisions are informed ones and that the choices you make are the ones that are right for you and your family.

According to Meg Taylor, a counsellor and herself an ex-midwife, the essential issue is one of control over the decision making. Women who feel that they have been consulted and who have had their wishes acknowledged are more likely to be satisfied with the experience and with their baby, than those who feel they were out of control of events and had things done to them. 'Participation in the decisions makes women feel that they have been consulted,' she says. 'When they don't have control over events, they may find they have very neg-ative feelings and thoughts afterwards, whereas that aspect of con-sultation leads to a much more positive view of the whole thing'.

Alison's story

Alison was expecting her baby at Christmas and she wasn't about to sacrifice her social life for that!

We had a major girls' night out planned for the 21st. I'd had twinges all day, but I wasn't going to let a little thing like that stop me. The twinges disappeared during the evening, and I had a lovely time — I got home about 2am. I was woken at 6am, with a heavy twinge, which I managed to persuade myself hadn't happened. Ten minutes later, I was forced to admit it probably had. I pottered about and had a shower, then put the TENS machine on. It worked brilliantly; I'd used it before, so I knew it was good. Concentrating on it, and having something to do, pressing the buttons and turning up the frequencies, really helped as well! I started it on low, which was enough to give me a tingly feeling in my back. I found it really took the edge off the pain.

About 1pm I called my midwife to tell her I was ready to go in and she said she'd meet me there. Of course the contractions stopped on the journey, and I was concerned it would all be a false alarm, but I needn't have worried. They came back with a vengeance when we got there. At 2.30pm, I was 4cm dilated and delighted to be certain that I was in labour. The TENS was working really well and I was happy just to wander around in my room till about 4.30pm when we went along to the birthing room. I carried on breathing through the contractions; I was so excited, but at the same time quite scared that it was all going to take hours yet. Last time, at the same point I'd needed intervention and I really didn't want all that again. About 5.45pm, I started to use the entonox. I don't think I'd used it properly the last time because this time I realised that if I took great big breaths and started as soon as I felt the first tightening, it was brilliant. It worked so well.

About 6.30pm, I had this huge pushing urge. I felt cold, and frightened that I wasn't ready, but my midwife pointed out that as she could already see the head, I probably was. Three pushes later, Tegan was born. I was overwhelmed, amazed, speechless with joy and triumph. It had been so easy — it was magic.

Dawn's story

When Dawn was expecting her first baby, she was happy to be advised by the professionals when she went into labour. She would have, she thought, whatever was recommended. She says, 'I had no thoughts about pain relief, really. I'd have what was suggested and go with the flow.'

In the event, Dawn was admitted to hospital on her due date because of high blood pressure. A week later, she went into labour on her own, just before she was supposed to be induced.

I had the pains in my back and down my legs. I know now it was because the baby was in an OP position, but at the time the back pain was awful. I was awake all night and when they examined me at about four in the morning I was 4 cm dilated, so they sent me down to the labour ward. I'd had no sleep, so I was given pethidine as soon as I got there, because I was so tired. I promptly fell asleep.

They were really busy and there wasn't a midwife I knew there, so they called my mum and my friend about 5 am to come and be with me. I felt so weird! I kept waking and sleeping, it was as if I was watching it all from another place and not really there at all. I kept saying odd things, like I thought my mum had some white trainers in her bag — I told her to take them home and wash them! Another time, I could smell nectarines so strongly, I asked for them to be taken out of my room, but there weren't any there at all.

After a while, I couldn't cope, so they tried to give me entonox, but it made me sick. I remember that, but a lot of it is really blurry. I remember being recommended to have an epidural, partly because of my blood pressure and partly because of the pain. It was such a relief to be pain-free and I remember it taking hardly any time at all. There was just a pressure in my back and that was it.

When I felt like pushing, I just felt so isolated from the event and even now I can't remember it properly. I kept falling asleep! Waiting for Lauren to scream seemed to take hours, but it was really only seconds. I was so relieved. My main feeling was one of relief, really. I thought, She's OK, I'm OK, I can sleep now. After the birth, everything seemed to take so long – waiting for her to cry, waiting to be stitched and all the time I was so tired.

When I got pregnant this time, I decided that my only plan was that I wasn't going to have pethidine again. I thought I'd rather have an epidural, because I was scared that the entonox would make me sick again. This time was great though. I had my own midwife, which made a huge difference, and when I was about 5 cm, she said to me, go on, try the gas and air. I did and it worked brilliantly. I used it right up till she was born two hours later and I wasn't sick at all! I kept as mobile as I could, even though the slightest movement brought on a contraction and Nicole was born with just two pushes. It was unbelievable!

I was in control this time – I was there! Making the decisions felt so much better. There won't be any more babies for us, so I'm really pleased it all went so well. I know the second time is easier, but it wasn't just easier, it was better. As my midwife said – it was textbook!

Jane's story

Jane was more sure of what she didn't want in the way of pain relief than of what she did! She wanted to have pethidine if she needed anything. 'I really felt I didn't want an epidural; I wanted to try and cope by myself, but I thought that the pethidine would take the edge off it.' Jane went into labour early on Christmas morning and used her TENS machine to help over the first hours.

I found it helped with the mild contractions, but when the real ones started later that night, it wasn't so good. By 2.30 am on Boxing Day, they were powerful, so we went into hospital. I spent the first three hours in the bath, with Till counting through the contractions – in German! – like a chant. It was brilliant! I'd worked so hard and was so tired, but when the midwife examined me at 7 am, I was only 1–2 cm dilated. The baby was in an OP lie and that was why it was taking so long and why I had all the pain in my back. I was devastated – really fed up.

They left us alone for a while, but about 11 am, Till had to go home for a while, because the cats needed sorting out, and he had to change his contact lenses. Once he'd gone, though, I found it really difficult to cope and at that point I asked for some pethidine. The midwife asked me if I wanted to wait until he came back but I said no; I'd said to him that his job was to make me stick to my birth plan and ask me if I'd changed my mind. I didn't want to be talked out of it!

If I'd known then that pethidine is a sedative, not an analgesic, I might have done things differently, but the back pain was so awful, I felt I had to have something. I remember expecting the pain relief to 'kick in' but it didn't. I just started to feel woozy. I could still feel all the contractions and I was so disappointed that it didn't work better. I really hated being on my own, and I would have loved to have had a midwife I knew with me. I didn't necessarily want someone to do something, I just wanted them to potter about and make soothing noises to me, like my mum used to when I was little and ill.

Then I started to use the entonox, because I couldn't breathe through the con-

tractions any more and I was starting to panic. It did help, and at least it gave me something to do. The pain was so strong, I used the mask as a talisman — I was afraid to let it go in case the pain got even worse. At about 5 cm dilated, the midwife gave me another dose of pethidine and I don't remember anything, except the contractions, until they said I could push. The problem was, I was so out of it that I couldn't seem to push properly. Eventually, after having a drip to get the contractions going again and the threat of forceps, I suddenly got an incredible pushing urge and managed to get her out by myself. We were over the moon with this little wriggly thing. I thought all I wanted to do was to sleep, but actually I stayed awake all night, just watching her.

There's just one more thing. After Josie was born she was very sleepy, and didn't want to feed. I know now that pethidine can affect babies in this way for up to three days afterwards. We persevered and succeeded, but she did have to have a bottle on her first day, which I hadn't wanted. Next time, I'll stick with the entonox!

Sue's story

Sue was keen to use alternative methods of pain relief. She says, 'I had an open mind about it all, really. I'm not the world's bravest person – my pain threshold, I would have said, was zero! – so I read a lot.'

I don't think I had any preconceived ideas, but I didn't like the thought of an epidural, and I don't think I would have liked to have a mask over my face. I'd also read somewhere that having a midwife you know reduces the need for pain relief, so I definitely wanted to know the midwife. That was the starting point and how I came to the Centre. I felt it was so important that I put my baby and myself in trusted hands, that it was a personal relationship. I finally decided that I would like to use a pool, as the idea of being supported in warm water appealed so strongly.

I was extremely fortunate in that my GP offered hypnotherapy for pain relief, but I didn't really think about it until I was about five months. Then, when I went, I wished I'd gone earlier. It was wonderful. It was the best excuse for half an hour a week, just lying around relaxing.

In the morning of my due date, I had period-like pains. I felt uncomfortable and restless, so I decided to have a bath, but I just couldn't relax. I put the hypnotherapy tape on and that calmed me down, because I had been feeling so edgy. Feeling much calmer, I went back to the bathroom and my waters broke!

All of a sudden, the contractions started coming every five minutes. Patrick phoned my midwife and I started to panic, then – I thought, this must be it, but it was all going so quickly and I was frightened about not making it in time. Poor Patrick was running about, getting everything in the car, but I did have a respite on the journey. We played the tape in the car, I focused on a picture of my cat and concentrated on that. I don't remember much about the journey till we got to the Centre, but once I saw my midwife, I just relaxed. There was a tremendous sense of relief and release and I felt I could just get on with it. It was going to be OK.

When we got in, my midwife examined me. I was so delighted to find I was 7 cm dilated and could get in the pool. The relief was wonderful! All the weight was lifted off me, I felt surrounded in the gentlest and most supportive of cuddles. It was so warm and free. Patrick leaned over the edge and supported my head and neck, which was wonderful for me, but his back was very stiff and uncomfortable next day; I'd recommend careful positioning for birth supporters! (The next time we got it right – Patrick got in the pool with me!)

Quite soon I got the urge to push, and again, the water really helped, as I could lean into it and didn't have to fight gravity. I felt weightless and so in control; it gave me something to push against.

I was scared when I was pushing – I felt so ambivalent. I wanted the baby out, but I didn't want it to hurt. You think to yourself, 'I can't do this', but you just have to. All that loving encouragement, from Patrick and my midwife made all the difference. I hadn't wanted to touch the baby's head, but once it was all out, I felt utter disbelief. "Oh, it is a baby!" I was so overwhelmed; I didn't know who she was, but she was mine. I was so triumphant, Patrick was in tears as we picked her up out of the water. I remember my midwife making us look and see what sex the baby was – it was such a wonderful, wonderful moment. Relief and disbelief which defy description.

Looking back on it all, I knew it was going to hurt and I had to accept that. I had to get on with it and get over it. It was all worth it, because of what I got. It only takes a short space of time, just a day out of your life, really. Being positive about it makes all the difference; your attitude to pregnancy and labour sets you up for afterwards.

Helen's story

The experience was on the whole very much as I expected. My mother had all of us at home and I've always had a view of childbirth as essentially normal. My work as a midwife has taken me all over the world and I can remember when I first worked in hospitals where an epidural service wasn't available, I couldn't believe it. It gradually dawned on me, though, that women are strong enough — they just get on with it. When I was in Hong Kong, the Nepalese women sometimes used to just have the babies quietly in the bathroom, because they didn't like to bother the midwife! It put things in perspective for me.

Continuity of care was very important to me and at the beginning, my community midwife was able to offer me just the care I wanted, even agreeing to go on call for me. It all changed later on though, when the Trust told her that she couldn't do any overtime or go on call for women, and I realised that I could be looked after by any one of up to twenty midwives, some of whom I'd never set eyes on. Luckily, I was able to find a midwife who was able to assure me of that continuity and she took over the responsibility for my care.

This belief in the normality of birth, when I knew my baby was in a back-to-back position (OP), enabled me to feel that I could resist the efforts of other professionals to persuade me to have an epidural, because I just felt sure it would be OK. My pregnancy was great and everything went well, but I must admit, when I went over my dates, I felt anxious about the possibility of an induction. I wanted to be able to negotiate and not to just accept a date because it was policy. In the event, I went into labour thirteen days past my date, so it was fine.

I was a bit anxious about the labour and tried hard to prepare myself — ignorance might have been bliss! — but in the event it wasn't as long or as bad as I thought it might be. I found the whole labour weird — I felt very detached from it. I could hear me talking to myself, with lots of positive propaganda, as if I were a midwife looking after me! I remembered all the advice and words of comfort I would use and gave them to myself. It was very peculiar when, late in first stage, I heard somebody grunting and realised it was me!

I never felt panicky, only weary when it was all over. The whole thing reinforced my practice philosophy and I thought to myself, 'Oh, I've been doing it OK after all!', but I think it's given me more empathy. I also think I pay more attention to baby care, now — before, I was always more interested in their mothers. On the whole, I think it adds to your street cred.

Charlotte's story

It was all really embarrassing and now, of course, my colleagues won't let me forget it. There can't be many midwives who get to 21 weeks without realising they're pregnant!

My cycle had been erratic since I came off the pill, so when I missed a period in July, I wondered if I might be pregnant. A test in September was negative and so were the two subsequent ones. A scan in October didn't show anything, although with hindsight, I was 4-6 weeks at this point. I'm on the big side, so the view wasn't all that good, but I just accepted it, and carried on.

I was a bit concerned about my lack of periods, so in January I had a chat with one of the doctors about it. She asked if I could be pregnant, but I laughed and said no. They were going to check my hormone levels and things, so I thought I'd better have a scan just to be certain. Oops — a twenty one week fetus!

Looking back, I had felt movements, but I thought they were wind and (this is really silly!) as soon as I found out, for two weeks I was sick in the mornings. I'd been envying a girl at work who was pregnant, then I found I was two weeks ahead of her!

Then I had to tell my husband, but I wanted to make it a bit more memorable than just saying, 'Guess what, I'm pregnant!', so I bought a card. The card said 'Love is a gift from God' and I signed it 'love from the baby'. It actually said Happy Anniversary as well, but I didn't see it. Anyway, he was totally confused, so I had to explain!

The baby was born on time, because I was induced due to my blood pressure rising. I blamed the hot weather, but everyone else said I looked bloated — even so, I wasn't worried. I'd gone along to the day unit to be checked out and they decided to keep me in for induction. I had two lots of prostin, then at about 2pm my friend, who was looking after me, broke my waters and I started properly.

I wanted an epidural, but because I couldn't keep still (I was contracting every

2–3 minutes), it didn't work very well, so I used gas and air as well. My husband was really quite worried, but I said to him, 'That's just the way it goes. It'll be OK'. I did everything wrong! I pushed when I shouldn't, I got my hands in the way – everything! Someone said to me that as a midwife, I should be more professional. I thought that was a terrible thing to say. I wasn't there as a midwife, I was a woman in labour, and that still rankles. Anyway, the baby was born at about 9.30pm and he was and is wonderful.

It's changed my practice completely, particularly with regard to breastfeeding. I really wanted to breastfeed, but he was always hungry – and he got colic – so very reluctantly I bottle-fed him. I felt as if the things I'd said to women just weren't always right and I learnt a lot about the baby blues when everything, happy or sad, makes you cry. I don't think midwives have to have had a baby, but it's made me more aware of what I say to women, because of what was said to me, and it's made me more understanding. I'd have another straight away if I could.

Louise's story

Before I'd even started midwifery, I'd made the decision to have my babies at home, so when I became pregnant in the last year of my training, I was determined to experience my pregnancy, birth and labour in the way I wanted.

In our area, we have a maternity centre, so I went to see the midwives there, as they are able to guarantee continuity of care wherever their clients want to deliver. I could have had my baby at the Centre, or with my midwife in hospital, but I had my heart set on a homebirth, so that was what I booked. My husband knew how I wanted to conduct my pregnancy and labour, but he found it hard to understand my reasons. In fact, when we first went to talk to my midwife, he sat there saying, 'Tell her, just tell her she can't have it at home'! Once he'd read some books and articles, however, he was as convinced as I was that this was the right thing to do. I had so much faith in my midwife, knowing she was happy to deliver me at home. We booked a birth pool and TENS for the labour.

I was actually due five days after my graduation day, which was a major event at Winchester Cathedral. I spent the whole day with my fingers crossed that my waters wouldn't break on stage! After the ceremony I began to notice the odd twinge. I told my midwife and, with hindsight, we both knew I was in early labour – Mark says, 'No-one told me!'

This suspicion was confirmed when, that evening, I had an overwhelming urge to clean the house from top to bottom. I'd done more housework in two hours than the previous two years ... The contractions built up until, at about 2am, we put the TENS on. We decided it was probably too early to fill the pool, but within half an hour I was out of control in my head, thinking that I'd only been in labour a couple of hours and I was acting like someone in transition. I coped by standing up, leaning on the edge of the pool and screaming.

When my midwife arrived, she was so reassuring and stopped me losing control by being so cheerful and calm. The water was brilliant, even though the boiler had turned itself off, and we had to use every utensil in the house to boil water! By 6.10am, I had to push, which I found frightening. Again my midwife calmed me down and she told me to go with the feelings and to do what I needed to do. When it came to it, nothing would have got me out of the pool, so Ella was born, slowly and gently, into the water about twenty minutes later.

The whole experience was so exhilarating. I can honestly say that I enjoyed it and felt that I could do it all over again that afternoon!

Mandy's story

Mandy's first baby, Samuel, was born by emergency Caesarean section, after she developed pre-eclampsia and was induced at 37 weeks. The whole thing just seemed to be out of her hands.

I felt such a failure. As if I'd been robbed.

When she became pregnant with her second child, she decided that she was going to be in charge. Mandy was told she would have to have an elective Caesarean, because of her previous section and because of her short stature. This wasn't what she wanted – she wanted to try to have her baby naturally, although she knew it might not work. Other options, such as an induction of labour, were not recommended, so Mandy went to an independent midwife who would support her in her wish to try for a homebirth, as she felt that at home, she could have her best shot at an intervention-free labour.

Mandy also felt strongly that she wanted to know the midwife who was going to be there at the birth, and to have built a relationship with her.

This time I felt so much stronger, knowing Ann. She would always explain things – if she said don't worry, I knew there was nothing to worry about!

Ann's confidence in birth as a normal process helped Mandy enormously. Even though she knew things might not go according to plan, she and Ann discussed the options and Mandy was able to bear those choices in mind. Alex, Mandy's husband, was completely supportive of her decision, even though he was very firm that he was not persuading her either way.

He said, this is your choice – I don't want you blaming me for it!

In the event, Mandy started contracting in the small hours, but by 9pm, it was clear that labour was not progressing – much the same as last time. The difference this time was that Mandy made her choice from the options that Ann gave her and decided to go into hospital. When they got there, Mandy decided to have an epidural and to wait until she was pain-free before deciding what to do.

I didn't want to be out of control. If they put the drip in and it didn't work, I'd still have to have the section, and I just didn't want to put her through what her brother went through.

Mandy's choice was to have another section – this time, though, she felt very sure that she was doing the right thing.

I felt I really had made the changes happen, rather than having them inflicted on me.

Her joy when baby Martha was lifted into the world, (at 3.2kg, a very good size for Mandy) was unbounded.

I really believed in myself and at least I felt I'd tried. Quite honestly, if we have another child, I'd try a vaginal birth again. It might not work, but I can make the decisions.

Fiona's story

Fiona is a firm believer in making your own decisions, which was particularly important to her when she was expecting her first baby.

When I thought about it beforehand, I suppose it was in a sort of rosy glow. I would control the pain, it would take me eighteen hours or so, I'd have a bit of gas and air. It would all be hunky-dory! Because I was so fit, I thought it would all be quite OK – a bit unrealistic, in retrospect!

Fiona started contracting on the Thursday.

I thought I'd have the baby on Friday. If I'd known it would take until Sunday lunch time, I don't know what I would have done. I contracted all Thursday night and all day Friday – every five minutes – so I got no sleep at all, and finally went into the hospital on Friday evening. As I was put on the antenatal ward, Steve had to go, so I was all alone, contracting every ten minutes or so. There was no-one to talk to or to be with, and I've never felt so alone. I was so pleased to see Steve on Saturday morning, but I was absolutely exhausted. We walked the ward all day on Saturday, and they wouldn't examine me because I wasn't in established labour, and I really wanted to know how I was doing.

Finally, about 5pm, Fiona insisted that she was examined. She was devastated to find she was only 2cm dilated.

The baby was posterior and so all the pain was in my back. Because I was so tired, I think, they took pity on me and gave me some pethidine which sent me off to sleep for two or three hours. I don't remember much about it – I was up on the ceiling, I think! – but when I woke up, I wanted to go to the loo. I just couldn't go though, so they had to catheterise me. I do wish I'd had a midwife with me that knew me. The night I was on my own, I was terrified, I couldn't pee, I hadn't slept for days – it was awful. I didn't know the midwives and they didn't know me. They didn't know I'd been brave and in control for days. They just saw this hysterical, demanding woman.

That was the last straw. I made a huge fuss and demanded an epidural. I'd been told I couldn't have one because I was only in early labour and it would knock off the contractions. I made such a to-do, that they went and woke up the poor anaesthetist at 3am and I got my epidural. It was such a relief! It did stop the contractions though, so I then had to have a drip and about 11am on Sunday they said I could push. The midwife told me when to push, but after an hour he still wasn't moving much. They suggested a ventouse, which worked really well. When he was born he had his hand up by his face, which was why he wouldn't come on his own.

Fiona says that, for a while after Ewan's birth, she was distressed. It had all been so different from her dream, but, she says positively, she's got it into perspective now.

I feel confident that it will be different next time. I'm glad it was me that made the choices. And, I know I can handle anything after that!

Sue's story

Sue's experience of labour was also very different from her dream. She had planned to have her baby in a birth centre, using a pool.

I thought it would be wonderful. This was our first baby and I'd set my heart on a waterbirth. I remember that I'd anticipated calm tranquillity, wandering around with Kim, then slipping into the water.

As the days passed after Sue's due date, however, she came under increasing pressure to have her labour induced. At fourteen days over her date, she discussed the situation with Kim and with her midwife, who had been caring for her throughout her pregnancy. Having agonised over the decision, she finally decided to go ahead with the induction, partly because she was tired of being pregnant, but mostly because she was afraid that if 'something awful' happened, and she had refused, it would all be her fault.

The worst thing of all was being induced. I felt robbed, and so did Kim, of that moment of excitement – the call to say it's started, come home. Having to go into hospital and being all clinical just wasn't what we'd planned. The most noticeable thing was all the hustle – being moved from room to room, people everywhere and the noise!

Sue was given prostin to start labour, which was followed by a syntocinon drip.

The whole thing was so different from my plan – because I was on the drip and being monitored, I had to stay on the bed, and because I couldn't move around the contractions were awful. I decided that if all this was going to happen, then I wasn't going to be heroic, and asked for an epidural. I never did get to use the pool!

Sue's midwife stayed with her throughout the labour, supporting and advising her.

What made it bearable was having my midwife there. We knew each other so well – she was sympathetic, she knew how I felt. She talked me through it, she was there for me, she was my resource – she was the interface between us and the hospital. Kim was great. He was my strength and I felt I had to be all right for him. He was so proud of himself for being there and so was I; he'd been frightened of the whole thing and he could have pulled out, but he didn't. He feels it's made a special bond between him and Charlotte. We made a terrific team between us.

Sue was very proud of the way she coped, even during the times when the epidural didn't work too well.

I kept thinking to myself, 'It'll be over soon'. I kept thinking that, all the way along, and just took things a chunk at a time, not thinking too far ahead. At the end of it, you know you're going to have a baby, so you focus on that.

After about eight hours of labour and an hour of pushing, it became obvious that both Sue and the baby were tired. At first, a ventouse was tried, but when that didn't shift the baby, the doctor decided to use forceps and baby Charlotte arrived, to tears of delight from both parents and the midwife! As Charlotte was over 9 pounds, Sue felt quite stunned by her achievement and says that, afterwards, she never felt so good.

I feel I could do it all again tomorrow, mostly because of what I got at the end! The overwhelming pride and triumph, the feeling of 'Look what I've done!' The pleasure you get from having done it and triumphed over it. I feel so very proud of myself. I won the marathon, I overcame everything.

None of it was anything like I'd planned, but once I held her, I didn't care. Next time, I won't look for the perfect birth. I would accept it for what it is, and take what comes. That's how it goes!

Appendix 1

The Midwives Information and Resource Service (MIDIRS)

MIDIRS is an organisation which provides midwives with a variety of useful information, including books, leaflets and a reference searching service.

The MIDIRS Informed Choice Leaflets

MIDIRS produce two series of leaflets which are aimed at both healthcare professionals and pregnant women. The leaflets are designed to help women to make informed choices during pregnancy, and are the result of a collaboration between MIDIRS and the NHS Centre for Reviews and Dissemination. The leaflets are supported by the Royal College of Midwives, the Royal College of Obstetricians and Gynaecologists and the Royal College of General Practitioners.

Series 1
Support in labour
Fetal heart rate monitoring in labour
Ultrasound screening in first half of pregnancy
Alcohol and pregnancy
Positions in labour and delivery

Series 2
Epidurals for pain relief in labour
Breastfeeding or bottle feeding
Antenatal screening for congenital abnormalities
Breech presentation – options for care
Place of birth

To purchase these leaflets, contact MIDIRS on FREEPHONE 0800 581009.

The MIDIRS Enquiry Service

The MIDIRS enquiry service is primarily aimed at midwives, but can provide up-to-date information on a wide range of midwifery and maternity care subjects. The MIDIRS database was set up in 1987 and now contains over 62,000 records, including articles from midwifery, nursing and medical journals, government reports, newspaper articles, books, chapters and leaflets. For a small fee you can order a 'standard search' from a list of over 350 popular subjects, including the following:

Social support in pregnancy (P30)
Childhood sexual abuse and effect on pregnancy (P65)
Midwife led care (M28)
Amniotomy (L1)
Nutrition and hydration in labour (L7)
Position and ambulation in labour (L13)
Pushing and bearing down (L15)
Third stage management (L19)
Induction of labour (L24)
Support/company in labour (L25)
Intermittent auscultation versus continuous fetal monitoring (L40)
Caesarean section – rates, increase, trends (L45)

You will receive a list of relevant documents, each with a brief summary attached. You can then contact MIDIRS to purchase full copies of any of the items that you would like to read.

For full information about the MIDIRS service, contact:

MIDIRS, 9 Elmdale Road, Clifton, Bristol BS8 1SL
Freephone 0800 581009
E-mail: midirs@dial.pipex.com
Website: http://www.midirs.org

Appendix 2

References and further reading

Chapter 3

Campbell, R. (1997). Place of birth reconsidered. In *Midwifery Practice: Core Topics 2* (J. Alexander, V. Levy and C. Roth, eds) pp. 1–22. Macmillan Press.

Campbell, R. and Macfarlane, A. (1994). *Where to be Born? The Debate and the Evidence*, 2nd edition. NPEU, Radcliffe Infirmary, Oxford.

Garcia, J. (1995). How well do the different ways of organizing midwifery services work? *Changing Childbirth Update*, no. 2, 6–7.

Green, J. M., Curtis, P., Price, H. *et al.* (1998). *Continuing to Care*. Butterworth-Heinemann.

Macvicar, J., Dobbie, G., Owen-Johnstone, L. *et al.* (1993) Simulated home delivery in hospital: a randomised controlled trial. *British Journal of Obstetrics and Gynaecology*, **100**, 316–323.

MIDRS (1999). *Midwife Led Care (M28)*. June. Midwives Information and Resource Service.

NHS Management Executive (1993). *A Study of Midwife and GP-led Maternity Units*. Department of Health, NHS Management Executive.

Shields, N., Turnbull, D., Reid, M. *et al.* (1998). Satisfaction with midwife-managed care in different time periods: a randomised controlled trial of 1299 women. *Midwifery*, **14**, 85–93.

Zander, L. and Chamberlain, G. (1999). ABC of labour care: place of birth. *BMJ*, **318**, 721–723.

Chapter 4

Clark, A. (1997). Getting the support you deserve. *Birthplace*, no. 61, 38–39.

Hodnett, E. D. (1998). *Caregiver Support for Women During Childbirth*. The Cochrane Library.

Gagnon, A. J., Waghorn, K. and Covell, C. (1997). A randomized trial of one-to-one nurse support of women in labor. *Birth*, **24**, 71–77.

MIDRS (1999). *Support/Company in Labour (L25)*. June. Midwives Information and Resource Service.

Moore, S. (1997). Psychological support during labour. In *Essential Midwifery* (C. Henderson and K. Jones, eds) pp. 219–227.

Parish, B. M. (1997). Review: professional support during labour improved labour outcomes. *Evidence-based Medicine*, **2**, 84.

Odent, M. (1996). Why laboring women don't need 'support'. *Mothering*, no. 80, 47–51.

Stansfield, P. (1997). An ancient tradition revived. *New Generation*, **16**, 8.

Walters, D. and Kirkham, M. J. (1997). Support and control in labour: doulas and midwives. In *Reflections on Midwifery* (M. J. Kirkham and E. R. Perkins, eds) pp. 96–113. Bailliere Tindall.

Watkins, T. M. (1998). Defining women's preferences for support during labor: a review of the literature. *Journal of Perinatal Education*, **7**, 9–16.

Chapter 5

Anderson, T. (1999). Hands/knees posture in late pregnancy or labour for malposition (lateral or posterior) of the presenting part. *Practising Midwife*, **2**, 10–11.

Baker, C. (1996). Nutrition and hydration in labour. *British Journal of Midwifery*, **4**, 568–572.

Beckwith, J. (1995). Lock up your monitors. *MIDIRS Midwifery Digest*, **5**, 441–443.

Berry, H. (1997). Feast or famine? Oral intake during labour: current evidence and practice. *British Journal of Midwifery*, **5**, 413–417.

Duffin, G. (1996). What is normal labour? *Midwifery Matters*, no. 69, 4–5.

Fraser, W. D., Krauss, I., Brisson-Carrol, G. *et al.* (1995). *Amniotomy for Shortening Spontaneous Labour*. The Cochrane Library.

Goffinet, F., Fraser, W., Marcoux, S. *et al.* (1997). Early amniotomy increases the frequency of fetal heart rate abnormalities. *British*

Journal of Obstetrics and Gynaecology, **104**, 548–553.

Henty, D. (1998). Brought to bed: a critical look at birthing positions. *RCM Midwives Journal*, **1**, 310–313.

MIDRS (1999). *Amniotomy (L1)*. June. Midwives Information and Resource Service.

MIDRS (1999). *Childhood Sexual Abuse and Effect on Pregnancy (P65)*. June. Midwives Information and Resource Service.

MIDRS (1999). *Intermittent Auscultation Versus Continuous Fetal Monitoring (L40)*. June. Midwives Information and Resource Service.

MIDRS (1999). *Nutrition and Hydration in Labour (L7)*. June. Midwives Information and Resource Service.

MIDRS (1999). *Position and Ambulation in Labour (L13)*. June. Midwives Information and Resource Service.

Oliver, S. and Needham, G. (1997). Appraising a randomized-controlled trial to enable informed choice. *British Journal of Midwifery*, **5**, 228–231.

Peterson, L. and Besuner, P. (1997). Positioning during the second stage of labor: moving back to basics. *Journal of Obstetric, Gynecologic and Neonatal Nursing*, **26**, 727–734.

Phoenix, E. (1996). No shame in survival. *International Journal of Childbirth Education*, **11**, 28–30.

Practising Midwife (1998). Eating and drinking in labour (I). A summary of medical research to facilitate informed choice about the care of mother and baby. *Practising Midwife*, **1**, 34–37.

Rhodes, N. and Hutchinson, S. (1994). Labor experiences of childhood sexual abuse survivors. *Birth*, **21**, 213–220.

Rosser, J. (1998). Continuous electronic fetal heart monitoring during labour. *Practising Midwife*, **1**, 60–61.

Rosser, J. and Anderson, T. (1998). Amniotomy to shorten spontaneous labour. *Practising Midwife*, **1**, 10–11.

Royal College of Midwives (1998). *Feeding not Fasting*. Royal College of Midwives.

Scutton, M., Lowy, C., O'Sullivan, G. (1996). Eating in labour: an assessment of the risks and benefits. *International Journal of Obstetric Anesthesia*, **5**, 214–215.

Sharp, D. A. (1997). Restriction of oral intake for women in labour. *British Journal of Midwifery*, **5**, 408–412.

Smith, M. (1998). Childbirth in women with a history of sexual abuse (I). A case history approach. *Practising Midwife*, **1**, 20–23.

Smith, M. (1998). Childbirth in women with a history of sexual abuse (II). A case history approach. *Practising Midwife*, **1**, 23–27.

Smith, M. (1998). Childbirth in women with a history of sexual abuse (III). A case history approach. *Practising Midwife*, **1**, 38–40.

Tallman, N. and Hering, C. (1998). Child abuse and its effects on birth: new research. *Midwifery Today*, no. 45, 19–21, 67.

Thacker, S. B. and Stroup, D. F. (1996). *Continuous Electronic Heart Rate Versus Intermittent Auscultation for Assessment during Labor*. The Cochrane Library.

Walsh, D. (1998). Birth positions in a large consultant unit: encouraging trends. *Practising Midwife*, **1**, 34–35.

Chapter 7

Bates, C. (1998). Rising caesarean section rates. *British Journal of Midwifery*, **6**, 204.

Chamberlain, G. and Zander, L. (1999). ABC of labour care: induction. *BMJ*, **318**, 995–998.

General Practitioner (1998). Behind the headlines. The caesarean dilemma. *General Practitioner*, **4**, 35.

Grant, J. M. (1999). Surgical and psychological experiences of caesarean section. *British Journal of Obstetrics and Gynaecology*, **106**, vii–viii.

Kristensen, M.O, Hedegaard, M. and Secher, N. J. (1998). Can the use of cesarean section be regulated? A review of methods and results. *Acta Obstetricia et Gynecologica Scandinavica*, **77**, 951–960.

Leitch, C. R. and Walker, J. J. (1998). The rise in caesarean section rate: the same indications but a lower threshold. *British Journal of Obstetrics and Gynaecology*, **105**, 621–626.

MIDRS (1999). *Caesarean Section – Rates, Increase, Trends (L45)*. June. Midwives Information and Resource Service.

MIDRS (1999). *Induction of Labour (L24)*. June. Midwives Information and Resource Service.

Oteri, O. and Tasker, M. (1997). Get set, and go: conventional action. *New Generation*, **4**, 11–12.

Simpson, K. R. and Poole, J. H. (1998). Labor induction and augmentation: knowing when, and how, to assist women in labor. *AWHONN Lifelines*, **2**, 39–42.

Stapleton, H., Tiran, D., Yelland, S. *et al.* (1997). Get set and go: complementary choices. *New Generation*, **16**, 11–12.

Stirrat, G. M. (1998). The place of caesarean section. *Contemporary Reviews in Obstetrics and Gynecology*, **10**, 177–184.

Summers, L. (1997). Methods of cervical ripening and labor induction. *Journal of Nurse-Midwifery*, **42**, 71–85.

Thorp, J. A. (1998). Epidural analgesia for labor: effect on the cesarean birth rate. *Clinical Obstetrics and Gynecology*, **41**, 449–460.

Chapter 8

Anderson, T. (1999). Active versus expectant management of the third stage of labour. *Practising Midwife*, **2**, 10–11.

Cruttenden, J. (1995). To push or not to push? *Modern Midwife*, **5**, 31–32.

Davis, G. (1997). Pushing: a spectator sport? *New Zealand College of Midwives Journal*, no. 17, 17–18.

d'Entremont (1996). Directed pushing in the second stage of labour. *Modern Midwife*, **6**, 12–16.

Downe, S. (1997). Changing times: practice and practicalities. *British Journal of Midwifery*, **5**, 629.

Featherstone, I. E. (1999). Physiological third stage of labour. *British Journal of Midwifery*, **7**, 216–221.

Halta, V. E. (1998). Taking the fear out of the third stage. *Midwifery Today*, no. 48, 18–22.

MIDRS (1999). *Pushing and Bearing Down (L15)*. June. Midwives Information and Resource Service.

Odent, M. (1998). Don't manage the third stage of labour! *Practising Midwife*, **1**, 31–33.

Sutton, J. (1997/98). A physiological second stage of birth without active pushing. *AIMS Journal*, **9**, 17–18.

Thompson, T. (1997). The second stage of labour: whose urge to push? *New Zealand College of Midwives Journal*, no. 16, 25–26.

Welford, H. (1997). When push comes to shove. *Independent Tabloid*, 8 May, 10–11.

Wood, J. and Rogers, J. (1997). The third stage of labour. In *Midwifery Practice: Core Topics 2* (J. Alexander, V. Levy and C. Roth, eds) pp. 113–126. Macmillan Press.

Index

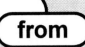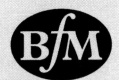
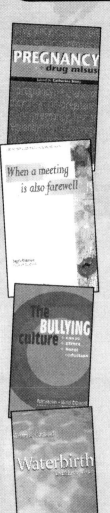